SUPER
CLEANSE

DETOX YOUR BODY FOR

LONG-LASTING HEALTH AND BEAUTY

SUPER CLEANSE

REVISED EDITION

ADINA NIEMEROW

WITH DIANA JASON WIGGETT

WILLIAM MORROW
An Imprint of HarperCollinsPublishers

SUPER CLEANSE REVISED EDITION. Copyright © 2008, 2012 by Adina Niemerow. All rights reserved. Printed in the United States of America. No part of this book may be used or reproduced in any manner whatsoever without written permission except in the case of brief quotations embodied in critical articles and review. For information address Harper-Collins Publishers, 10 East 53rd Street, New York, NY 10022.

HarperCollins books may be purchased for educational, business, or sales promotional use. For information please write: Special Markets Department, HarperCollins Publishers, 10 East 53rd Street, New York, NY 10022.

FIRST WILLIAM MORROW PAPERBACK EDITION PUBLISHED 2012.

Designed by Jessica Shatan Heslin/Studio Shatan, Inc.

The Library of Congress has catalogued the previous edition as follows:
Niemerow, Adina.
    Super cleanse: detox your body for long-lasting health and beauty/Adina Niemerow with Diana Jason.—1st ed.
        p.   cm.
    Includes bibliographical references and index.
    ISBN 978-0-06-137458-6 (alk. paper)
    1. Detoxification (Health)   I. Jason, Diana.   II. Title.

RA784.5.N54 2008
613—dc22

2008010501

ISBN 978-0-06-211336-8 (pbk.)

12   13   14   15   16   WBC/RRD   10   9   8   7   6   5   4   3   2   1

I dedicate this book to all the people reconnecting with the power of earth medicine.

CONTENTS

Seven Essentials of Your Daily Routine ▪ 19

The One-Day Wonder Cleanse ▪ 29

The Winter Wake-Up Cleanse (5 to 7 Days) ▪ 169

The Green Buzz Cleanse (5 to 7 Days) ▪ 181

End on a High Note ■ 233

ACKNOWLEDGMENTS

This book is an accumulation of all the inspiration and information shared by my amazing teachers and mentors, including: my instructors at the Heartwood Institute, especially Paul Pitchford, author of *Healing with Whole Foods,* and Bruce Burger, author of *Esoteric Anatomy*; the instructors and staff at the Natural Gourmet Cookery School in New York City; Dr. David Jubb of Jubb's Longevity in New York City; Dr. Gabriel Cousens, author and founder of the Tree of Life Rejuvenation Center in Patagonia, Arizona; Kasha, Tim and Michella of the Tree of Life Café; Hillary Hitt of the Dharma Healing Center in Koh Samui, Thailand; Debra Reardon, Ayurvedic teacher and practitioner; Chef Juliano; and Thomas Keller for his culinary skill and magic in the kitchen. My life was transformed by your teachings and wisdom, and I thank you for the opportunities I had to study and work with you.

Writing a book can take over your life and I realized very quickly that I needed a partner to make the experience fun. Why do anything that you don't enjoy, right? This book became real with the help of Diana Jason. Diana, I was grateful every day for your selfless devotion of time, energy, creativity and support in helping me get my message clear and organized. I could not have asked for a better copilot over the past year. Special thanks to Oli Wiggett for sharing Diana with me.

I also want to acknowledge the following for granting permission for quotes and reproductions from their work: Donna F. Smith, PhD, ND, CCN; Dr. Gabriel Cousens, MD; and the Natural Gourmet Cookery School.

A host of other people helped bring this book to life by opening doors for me, testing recipes, providing testimonials, brainstorming ideas or sharing their expertise and advice with me. So, I send my thanks to: Judith Regan, Oz Garcia, Doug Childers, Brooke Asher, Sandy Vaughn, Jodi Simon, Brooke Turner Waterhouse, Dorothy Kinne, Shakti Kennedy, Holly Kopman, Jean Watson, Françoise Wiggett, Kelly Murdock, Loryn Herridge, Jennifer York, Jonny Leroy, Joe Conte, Justin Schmidt, Karen Lehner, Angela Hoxsey, Abbie Scianamblo, Elizabeth Eckholt, Mark Susnow, Meredith Geller, Emily Ryan, Charity Tooze, Susan Ferrington, Marc Halprin, Theresa Vargo, Elisha Trotter Tucker, Adam Kahn, Karen Mondoux, Lori Hunter, and everyone at Café Gratitude in San Francisco.

I'm also grateful to Anne Cole and Cassie Jones, my editors, for their thoughtful insights, and to HarperCollins for giving me the opportunity to publish this book.

Last, but not least, I thank my family. Special thanks to Mom, Dad, Daryl, Daron, Aness Pogni, Jacob Steinlauf, and my love, Adam, for always being present for me and supporting my dreams. I am so blessed to have you in my life.

PREFACE

In the few years since this book was first published, I've been blessed with ongoing feedback from new readers and "repeat Super Cleansers." They've emailed and blogged to share their success stories about how cleansing has changed the way they eat for good, to ask questions, and to share critiques and ideas for making the cleanse experience easier. Based on all the feedback, I jumped at the opportunity to keep *Super Cleanse* current and get real about a few things, including the #1 reason most people try a cleanse, the rising cost of food, and the ways people are staying connected and informed in the world today. Here's how getting real plays out in this edition of the book:

First, the #1 reason most people take the leap into cleansing is *(drum roll, please . . .)* to lose weight. It's a fact that I didn't want to give in to in the first edition of the book, because—for me—cleansing is not a fad or crash diet, it's a window into the power of food as medicine and an opportunity to examine what you're consuming that may be undermining your health. But the people have spoken, and it was time to shift my thinking! So I created the Super Slim Down, a nutritional cleanse that's satisfying, chock-full o' nutrients, and carefully crafted not to include foods that weigh you down. You may come for the weight loss, but I'm betting you'll stay for the incredible impact eating well has on your entire being.

Next, I've simplified the recipes *and* made them easier on the wallet. I've given you other options for the more expensive or difficult-to-find ingredients, taken them out entirely, or replaced them with more economical alternatives.

Last, I can see how important it is to be connected, and how technology is transforming the way we communicate and create community. While I still firmly believe that we need to unplug on a regular basis to reconnect to the rhythms of nature, I also want to support you, so please reach out to me with feedback, questions, and ideas at adinaniemerow.com. I will post comments, testimonials and educational videos on my website to support your journey.

That, dear readers, is how I've freshened the book to make it even more appealing and easy for you to cleanse.

WHY CLEANSE?

Fasting and cleansing to purify the body and mind are not new concepts. They were first embraced thousands of years ago as a pathway to connect with the divine and achieve higher levels of awareness and clarity. It's more relevant than ever today.

I created the 10 cleanses in this book to awaken the spirit as much as the body and mind. They're mini retreats that pull you out of your daily routine so that you can examine what you're consuming—and what's consuming you—whether it's the food you eat, the lifestyle you choose or the environment you're living in. They give you a quick tune-up as well as an opportunity to recalibrate and realign with your internal guidance system.

So much of the food we choose to eat fogs our life force and weighs down the body in dis-ease. The effects are making headlines every day. Rates of heart disease, diabetes and cancer are on the rise, prescriptions for medications to treat depression and anxiety are at record levels, two out of three American adults are overweight, the rate of autoimmune disease is growing, chronic fatigue syndrome is a new fixture in our country's lexicon—and the list goes on and on.

Fortunately, we can set ourselves free from low energy, stress, illness, obesity, addiction, depression and a host of other physical, emotional or spiritual ailments we might be facing. The path back to wellness is simple—we just need to take a step out of our usual routine to reassess and understand how food and lifestyle choices are shaping our health.

For 17 years, I trekked across the globe exploring the healing powers of food. Along the way, I had the privilege to work with pioneers in the "food as medicine" movement. I cleansed, studied, cooked, sweat, prayed and meditated with holistic healers. I went out there looking for the "one answer" to naturally healing the body and found there isn't one right way. Staying in balance and being healthy is an evolution, and we can each start where we are. Doing a cleanse is a great first step.

My cleanses are hybrids of all that I've seen, experienced and learned. Food is definitely the anchor in each one, because what you eat affects your whole being. Preparing food from this book even one day a week will have a positive impact on how you feel—and everything in life is better when your body feels good.

We have the answer to staying clear, light and awake. So my question to you is: How can we not take time out to do a cleanse?

The revolution begins within.

HOW TO USE THIS BOOK

One size does not fit all when it comes to healing the body. Constitution, diet and lifestyle have a big influence on how ready people are to do a cleanse and how stringent a cleanse they can manage. Any number of factors play into the equation, including how well—or how poorly—they've been eating, their relationship with or addiction to foods, their current state of health, and the levels of stress in their daily lives.

Not everyone is prepared—physically, mentally or emotionally— to immediately jump into a rigorous detox, so I created a series of nine cleanses to fit different states of readiness—from gentle programs that slowly introduce a vegetarian diet to green-juice fasts that rapidly detox the body and flush the intestinal tract. As you dive into those chapters, you'll get a sense of which cleanse you feel ready for.

To be certain you understand what you're getting into, I urge you to read through the earlier sections in the book to get a handle on the cleansing process and learn what you can expect to see and feel.

I've tried to make this journey as smooth as possible for you by presenting the information in a lighthearted, easy-to-use and easy-to-understand way. To that end, this book includes a brief overview of the science behind cleansing and why it works, recipes that use readily available ingredients and require the minimum amount of equipment, hints and fun activities to help minimize the detox symptoms and boost the positive effects of the cleanses, and tactics to help you de-stress and regain your equilibrium.

Finally, there's information on how to break a cleanse and ease back into a wholesome, daily diet that nurtures your body, mind and spirit, so take time to understand the process and know what to expect before jumping in.

A few words of caution: Once you've picked a cleanse, check in with your physician or holistic health-care practitioner to see if it's right for you, considering preexisting conditions you may have or medications you may be taking. You may have a medical condition that makes cleansing unwise at this particular point in your life.

Also, know that the cleanses in this book are not ongoing maintenance diets; they're intended to be done for a limited number of days to help clean out your system and jump-start a new way of eating. The recipes are packed with enzymes, vitamins and minerals that clear your body, but they don't have the full complement of the nutrients your body needs in a long-term daily diet. So I've provided guidance on how long to follow each program and the maximum number of times a year to do it.

Now, if you're ready to learn about the miraculous healing power of a cleanse, read on!

SUPER
CLEANSE

THE NITTY-GRITTY
ON CLEANSING

Word on the Street: We Are What We Eat

Food is medicine—if we're choosing the right things to eat. Some of the food we put on our table may be undermining our health in ways we don't even realize. Many of the fruits and vegetables in our markets are sprayed with chemical fertilizers and pesticides, and most meats are pumped up with antibiotics, hormones or fungicides. When we ingest these chemicals, they can have a harmful effect on the body.

The problem with many of the foods we eat goes beyond the meat and produce departments. Just take a stroll through the rest of the grocery store and you'll see that most of what's stocking the shelves bears no resemblance to food grown on a farm. A lot of it has been processed—irradiated, bleached or heated—to the point that it's stripped of the life-giving enzymes, vitamins, fiber and minerals that our bodies need to thrive. Our bodies have a hard time digesting processed flours, sugars, oils and salts, so that food ends up clogging our intestines, severely impairing our bodies' ability to efficiently absorb nutrients and void waste.

To take responsibility for our health, we have to become more aware of the food we eat. We need to be detectives when it comes to reading food labels and learn how to identify the ingredients that undermine our health. Don't automatically trust a "natural" sticker that's been slapped on a package in the store. If we find out where our food comes from, we can better appreciate the importance of eating whole, organic foods.

Bottom line: Food that's grown wild on this Earth, that hasn't been genetically engineered, processed or tampered with, is good for us. Everything else is questionable.

THE DIRTY BAKER'S DOZEN

Eliminating the following things from our diets—even reducing our intake—can have a dramatic and positive impact on our health:

- Bleached, refined flours
- Refined sugars, high-fructose corn syrup
- Table salt
- Trans fats and refined oils (including processed corn, canola, sunflower, safflower and vegetable oils)
- Meats treated with hormones or antibiotics; farmed fish
- Foods sprayed with pesticides and herbicides
- Genetically modified foods
- Pasteurized dairy and GMO soy
- Additives such as preservatives, nitrates, and artificial flavorings and colorings
- Fast foods and fried foods
- Sodas and juices with added sugars
- Tap water
- Alcohol

Drop Acid

The Dirty Baker's Dozen (see the list at left)—especially in combination with stimulants such as caffeine, tobacco and drugs—elevate acid levels in our bodies. That's a problem, because health and disease are directly tied to pH levels in our system: When the body is in an acidic state, it stops functioning properly and disease can take root. So one important function of a cleanse is to bring the body's chemistry back into balance.

The 14-point pH scale measures the alkalinity or acidity of a solution—a pH level of 1 to 7 is considered acidic, and a pH level above 7 is considered alkaline. With the exception of the stomach, large intestine, skin and female reproductive organs, the rest of our organs and systems function optimally in a slightly alkaline state. If the body senses that any of its internal fluids (blood, lymphatic fluid, bile, cerebrospinal fluid, etc.) are too acidic, it takes action to restore an alkaline state. If our diets aren't providing the alkaline minerals required to restore balance in these fluids, the body will leach the minerals from our organs, muscles, ligaments and bones. The part of the body that has sacrificed those minerals then becomes acidic and vulnerable to illness.

To reduce acid levels in our system, we need to (1) reduce acid-forming foods from our diet; (2) clear acidic, undigested food from the intestines; (3) flush toxins from the body; (4) add alkaline foods and drinks to neutralize acidity; and (5) relax the body and mind. When we do that, we can reduce congestion, inflammation and pain throughout our bodies, invigorate ourselves, and increase our flexibility. We can get to a place where we're able to suck every juicy nutrient from the food we're eating and maintain an alkaline balance in the body.

DRUGS AND DIGESTION

Over-the-counter, prescription and recreational drugs drive up acid levels in the body. In addition, some drugs—such as antibiotics—kill the flora (good bacteria) in the intestine that aid in digestion, hindering our ability to break down the food we eat. When we eat an alkaline diet, it boosts our immunity and restores a state of balance in the body. Many people find they're less reliant on these acid-producing, digestion-unfriendly medications.

Acid or Alkaline?

A food can be acidic in its natural state but become alkaline when it's digested—and vice versa. That's because digestion oxidizes food—essentially burning it up. The by-product of that intestinal fire typically has a different acid or alkaline level from the food we've popped into our mouths. For instance, a lemon is acidic in its raw state. However, once eaten, it breaks down into carbon dioxide and water and leaves behind alkaline minerals such as sodium, potassium and calcium. On the other hand, animal products, such as meat or dairy products, can leave behind acidic compounds such as phosphates, sulfates and nitrates. See pages 217–218 for a chart listing the relative acidity or alkalinity of different foods.

Fresh juices and wheatgrass shots are great, quick ways to help alkalize the body. I've built green juices into the cleanses, but I encourage you to run in and grab a wheatgrass shot if you pass a juice bar.

An Acid State of Mind

There's more affecting our pH levels than the food we eat and stimulants or drugs we take. Our thoughts and feelings also play a big part in how acidic our body is. When we're stressed out, angry, unhappy, depressed or focused on negative thoughts, that actually increases the levels of acid in our body. On the flip side, when we're happy, relaxed, positive and at peace, we reduce our acid levels.

So an important part of a cleanse is taking time to unplug from our usual routines and making time for meditation to rest and clear our minds.

WHAT'S YOUR pH?

You can test your pH by buying pH strips at your local health-food store, but another option is to take note of any symptoms you may be experiencing. There are several telltale signs for how acidic or alkaline your body might be. Symptoms of being too acidic include stiff joints, arthritis, muscle tension, stress headaches, addiction to stimulants, itchy skin or acne, anger, a short temper, and chronic negative thoughts. Check in with yourself to see if your body is trying to tell you it's time to "drop acid."

Clear Your Body, Free Your Mind and Spirit

A good cleanse reboots our whole being. It provides a magnified awareness, a fresh perspective, spiritual renewal and physical rejuvenation. When we get rebalanced, we get clearer about who we are and who we're committed to being. That's the miraculous and healing power of a cleanse.

GET READY . . . GET SET . . .

To help you get prepared, here are some more details about the cleansing process and a few tricks of the trade to make doing a cleanse as easy as possible, including:

✳ Additional info on the healing reactions you may experience, to ready you for what you might feel and see

✳ Dietary and lifestyle suggestions for the week leading up to the cleanse

✳ A checklist for the week before you start cleansing

Laying the groundwork with the above should help you alleviate unnecessary stress and avoid any surprises while you cleanse.

NOTE: You may have a preexisting condition or be at a place in your life emotionally that would make it unwise to do a particular cleanse—or start any cleanse—at this time. For instance, individuals who are hypoglycemic, diabetic, mentally ill or recovering from surgery should not cleanse without clearance from a physician—and women who are pregnant or nursing should not cleanse. I highly recommend speaking with your physician or licensed health-care provider for guidance. On the basis of your needs and current state of health, they'll be able to advise you whether you should do a cleanse and which cleanse is right for you.

Healing Reactions in the Body

I mentioned healing reactions earlier in the book, but it's a point worth reiterating. Depending on your pre-cleanse diet and lifestyle, and how stringent a cleanse you choose, you may experience a spectrum of physical symptoms as the body purges toxins. They're an uncomfortable but normal part of detoxification, and they usually subside within the first two days. These symptoms may include:

* Mood swings, anger, impatience or depression
* Weakness
* Headaches
* Nausea
* Cramping, gas, diarrhea or constipation
* Hunger pangs
* Body or joint aches
* Wild dreams
* Skin rashes or acne
* Bad breath or a coating on the tongue
* Insomnia or fatigue

These side effects are generally more prominent with the more stringent cleanses, such as the Urban Revitalizer, Winter Wake-Up or Green Buzz, and less prominent in gentler cleanses, such as the Laughing Buddha, Karma or Three-Day Face-Lift. If you've had a fairly "clean" diet leading up to the cleanse, you might not experience any of these symptoms—lucky you!

Easing the Detox Process

Here are some dietary and lifestyle tips for the week leading up to the cleanse to help mellow the physical healing reactions you might experience:

* If you don't drink much water, start adding a few additional glasses of purified water to your daily routine.

* If you eat meat every day, cut it down to every other day.

* If you start your day with a cup or two of coffee, consider switching to drinks with chicory root, herbal teas or yerba mate tea.

* If you make pasta, rice or noodles with dinner, try substituting an additional vegetable or quinoa (quinoa is a seed that looks like couscous, but it's higher protein).

* If you regularly eat frozen or processed foods, consider making simple, fresh meals at home that week.

* If you smoke or drink alcohol, cut back on your daily intake so you're not going cold turkey during the cleanse. To help curb cravings for nicotine, drink ¼ cup of lobelia tea sweetened with licorice root, or drink 10 to 12 drops of lobelia tincture in a glass of water several times a day. Lobelia tea, licorice root and lobelia tincture can be found in local health-food stores.

If you're able to wean yourself from these things even a little bit, you'll have an easier time cleansing.

TO JAVA OR NOT TO JAVA . . . THAT IS THE QUESTION

Two of the first questions I get from clients when they begin a cleanse are "Do I really need to give up coffee?" and "Can I just drink decaf instead?" The answers are "Yes, you should," and "Please don't, it's just as bad." When we understand the effect of coffee on the body and what's in regular and decaffeinated coffee, we can see how they undermine the cleansing process and damage our bodies. Insights from Donna F. Smith, PhD, ND, CCN, shed light on the dark side of the dark-roast brew many of us love:

The Top Five Reasons for Kicking the Coffee Habit

1 Coffee sets off a chain reaction in the body that stresses the adrenals. The acid-based oil in coffee irritates the lining of the stomach and increases gastric acidity. That sparks the secretion of adrenaline by the body. Adrenaline stimulates insulin secretion, which fuels hypoglycemia (low blood sugar). The end results are tension, a mild rise in blood pressure, a craving for sweets 2 or 3 hours later, low energy and a depressed mood.

2 Coffee counteracts different medications. When our blood sugar drops, the body ups the production of epinephrine—which counteracts the medications typically prescribed for people suffering from pain, obesity, hypertension or depression.

3 Coffee causes nutritional deficiencies. Heavy coffee drinkers have a deficiency of the B_1 vitamin thiamine. Symptoms of B_1 deficiency range from fatigue, nervousness and malaise to aches, pains and headaches. In addition, regular consumption of coffee prevents nutrients from being absorbed effectively in your small intestines, which leads to further vitamin and mineral deficiencies.

4 Pesticides in coffee are toxic to the body. Coffee growers in Colombia—where a vast amount of our coffee comes from—often use harmful pesticides when growing their beans, such as aldrin, dieldrin, chlordane and heptachlor. Some scientists speculate that coffee beans are the most significant source of these toxins in U.S. diets.

5 Long-term coffee consumption taxes the liver, increasing toxicity in the body and opening the door to disease. The function of the liver is to filter the blood so that it can clean and nourish the cells in our body. When the liver gets overloaded trying to detoxify chemical residues in coffee (and the foods and other substances we bring into our bodies), it becomes congested. And when the liver is congested, it doesn't properly filter the blood. Impure blood ends up circulating through the body, impeding cells' ability to regenerate and grow healthy tissue.

Unfortunately, drinking decaffeinated coffee isn't any better than drinking regular coffee, because it can contain large concentrations of trichloroethylene—a chemical that's also used as a degreasing agent in the metal industry and a solvent and dry-cleaning agent in the clothing industry. Trichloroethylene is also related to vinyl chloride, a chemical in plastic that's been linked to certain types of liver cancer.

If you can't fathom getting through the day without that coffee taste, try herbal drinks with chicory, which has the flavor you love without the harmful side effects. If you need a pick-me-up to start the day, give yerba mate a try. It has effective stimulants but doesn't produce as many of the negative health effects that caffeine does. An even better, more healthful, option is herbal tea. Herbal teas seem weak to you? Pump them up by using two or three tea bags per cup of tea and letting them steep for a longer period of time. Add a bit of nut milk if you'd like to drink them latte-style (see recipe on page 93).

Healing Reactions in the Mind and Spirit

It's not uncommon to feel a heightened sense of clarity and focus after the first couple of days of a cleanse. Clients have described it to me as a fog lifting. The way around hurdles in life may become clearer, and the path to achieving goals may suddenly become apparent.

Journaling can be especially uplifting during this part of the process. In addition to helping you work through obstacles that may have been silently affecting your health and state of mind, the journal provides a chronicle of your progress—documenting what might ultimately be a testimonial of your road back to wellness. Ideally, you'll be able to reflect back on journal entries to stay focused on epiphanies or ideas you have during the cleanse and keep moving forward in a new, positive direction.

As our minds and bodies clear, doors can open to a more spiritual awakening as well. Eating clean, whole foods shifts vibrations in the body. Without toxicity dulling the spirit, we come alive inside again. With a heightened sense of serenity, calmness and balance, we can get to a place of quiet equilibrium and reconnect with our true nature, those around us and the Earth. For some of my clients, this spiritual side of cleansing is as profound as the shifts they feel in their mind and body.

ANGELA'S TESTIMONIAL

I'd been feeling the need to get off the caffeine merry-go-round and balance my energy somehow so that I could be more effective in my non-profit work, as well as my career and personal life. When I found out Adina was leading a cleanse at Café Gratitude, I signed right up—even though it meant an hour-and-a-half drive, each way, for five days.

During the cleanse I experienced a sense of release on every level—physically, emotionally and spiritually. I lost weight, which was great, but that wasn't the best part. By the fifth day, my values and purpose came into sharp relief. I was clear about my purpose to help heal the planet. My communications with other people became much more direct and loving as I began to feel more connected to everyone around me.

I'd never seen the connection between diet and the state of my relationships (as well as the state of the world) with so much clarity. And I realized that what I brought into my body and the lifestyle I chose were the keys to maintaining the level of clarity and peace I had found. It was an extremely intense but enjoyable learning experience that will influence the rest of my life.

A cleanse may start in the body, but it has the power to permeate your whole being. So I've built meditations, breathing exercises and mantras into different chapters to help spark holistic healing and a sense of reconnecting to spirit and the Earth.

Pre-cleanse Checklist

I based this to-do list for the week leading up to the cleanse on questions and comments from clients. Taking time to go through these steps in advance will help you select an appropriate cleanse, be sure you have everything on hand that you need to get started, and minimize the running around and common pitfalls ("Honey, who's feeding the kids?") that can increase stress during a cleanse.

- ✓ **Choose a cleanse.** Read through the cleanse chapters and select one that you think is right for you. Run that program by your physician to make sure you don't have a preexisting condition that would prevent you from doing that cleanse.

- ✓ **Learn the daily routine.** Read through the "Seven Essentials of Your Daily Routine" chapter (page 19) to get familiar with the daily activities that will ease the detox phase and help you get the most from your cleanse.

- ✓ **Plan time for yourself.** If you have vacation time available and can take time off during the cleanse, seriously consider doing that. If that's not a possibility, be sure to build time into your daily routine to practice the meditations, breathing exercises, mantras or other supportive disciplines included with the cleanse. Unplugging from your daily fast-paced routine will dramatically increase the positive effects of the cleanse.

✓ **Choose recipes.** To accommodate different palates, I put more recipes than the actual number of meals in several of the cleanse chapters, so read through the recipes and decide which you'd like to do when.

✓ **Make a shopping list** of the foods, supplements and equipment you might need to purchase. The goal is to eat food that's as fresh as possible. So, if you're doing a 5- or 7-day cleanse, buy the ingredients you'll need for the first few days and then do a second run to the store for the meals you'll eat later in the week.

✓ **Make appointments** for the supportive disciplines, if necessary. For instance, I recommend a hot–cold plunge in the Winter Wake-Up Cleanse, which requires a hydrotherapy or spa appointment. I suggest a facial massage for the Three-Day Face-Lift, which is typically done by a Shiatsu practitioner. And if you decide to go to a colon hydrotherapist, you can make that appointment in advance as well.

✓ **Recruit a friend.** I've found that doing a cleanse with a friend or two is great way to create a support team for yourself—you can share what you're experiencing, hold each other accountable for sticking with the cleanse as you detox and celebrate the progress you make together. You can share the work of making the recipes too!

✓ **Brief your partner.** If you have a partner, speak with him or her about your plans to do a cleanse, and ask for support. Explain the detox process and the fact that you could be feeling physically rough and emotionally raw for a few days. Your partner may need to cook for him- or herself while you cleanse, and cook for the kids if you have children. Who knows, your partner may decide to do the cleanse with you!

✓ **Reflect and set intentions.** Set aside some quiet time to think about why you're doing the cleanse and what you hope to achieve. Write these down in a journal and set intentions for what you'd like to see change in your post-cleanse life. When I ask clients to sit back and visualize what they're hoping to achieve—what's different, what does that feel like, what does that look like—they seem to have more success in getting there.

✓ **Be good to yourself the day before.** The day or night before a cleanse, I've had clients tell me they "went to town"—ate all the comfort foods they were going to miss during the week, stayed out late partying, and so on—not unlike the way many of us overindulge on New Year's Eve before our New Year's resolutions kick in the next day. That's not an uncommon response, but it could make the first day of cleansing that much harder. I recommend eating light, healthy meals, having a restful day, and getting to bed early the night before.

The Right Equipment

Each cleanse in this book includes a number of recipes for blended soups or smoothies and fresh juices, so you'll want to have a high-speed blender and a juicer on hand. Any high-speed blender will do the trick for the soups and smoothies, but picking a juicer—if you don't already have one—can be trickier. There are several different kinds of juicers out there, and the names alone can be confusing: centrifugal ejection, masticating, manual press, single-auger, dual-stage auger, and twin-gear press, to name a few.

My experience in kitchens and in working with clients has shown me that it ultimately comes down to what you'll be juicing, cost, how easy it is to use and clean, and the quality of the juice it produces.

My juice recipes are primarily vegetable-based. Because vegetables have tougher, more fibrous cell walls than fruit does, they require greater mechanical power to render the juice. That automatically narrows your list of options. Keeping that in mind—along with the desirable combination of cost, ease and juice quality—there are three types of juicers I recommend to my clients. They're described below, listed from least to most expensive.

NOTE: These recommendations are based on the recipes included in this book. If you want to be able to use your juicer to make all-fruit juices, sorbets, nut butters or baby food, these may not be the best machines for you. Check out the website *www.discountjuicers.com* for a wealth of information about what juicers are best for other functions.

Centrifugal Ejection Juicer

✳ **How it works:** As produce is pushed through the feeder tube, it hits a spinning shredder disk, releasing the juice into a strainer basket. The basket spins at a high rate of speed, forcing the juice through it. The pulp is ejected out of the side of the machine into a collection basket.

✳ **Brand worth considering:** Jack LaLanne.

✳ **Price point:** As low as $100 online.

✳ **Pros:** It's easy to use and easy to clean, and at a good price if you're not yet convinced you'll be making juices on a regular, post-cleanse basis.

✳ **Cons:** This type of juicer operates at higher rpm than the other two juicers, which has two main drawbacks. First, the higher rpm oxidizes the produce to a greater degree; once juice starts oxidizing, it begins losing nutrients. Second, this juicer is much louder than the other models.

Dual-Stage Single-Auger Juicers

✳ **How it works:** In stage 1, the juicer crushes the produce into the walls of the juicer, extracting some of the juice. The pulp then continues on to stage 2, in which it's pushed through a finer screen to pull out more of the juice.

✳ **Brands and models worth considering:** Solo Star II and the Omega 8003.

✳ **Price point:** As low as $219 online.

✳ **Pros:** Lower rpm translates into (1) less oxidation and thus a higher-quality, more nutrient-rich juice and (2) a quieter machine. I upgraded to a Solo Star II and have been very happy with it.

✳ **Cons:** They're more expensive and slightly harder to clean than the Jack LaLanne. (The Omega is easier to clean than the Solo Star, but it costs slightly more.)

Twin-Gear Press Juicer

✳ **How it works:** The produce is pushed through two gears that shred and then squeeze the pulp to render the juice.

✳ **Model worth considering:** Green Star

✳ **Price point:** As low as $399 online.

✳ **Pros:** The gears turn at a very low rpm, minimizing the oxidation of the juice. This model is ideal for people who want to go beyond juicing and make nut butters, sorbets, apple-sauces, and so on. Earlier versions of the Green Star were in some of the kitchens I worked in, and they were very versatile.

✳ **Cons:** Price; the manual pressure required to feed the fruits and vegetables into the machine, and the fact that these machines have the most pieces to clean after juicing.

Juicing Alternatives

If you aren't willing to invest in a juicer but still want to cleanse, you have two alternatives: You can find a local merchant or juice bar that makes fresh, organic green juices or you can try the blending method. To blend your juices, put the ingredients in a high-speed blender, add water to cover, blend until smooth and then strain them through a fine sieve or nut-milk bag. Keep in mind, however, that blending oxidizes the juice faster (neutralizing some of the beneficial enzymes), and pressing and straining the solids to remove the juices makes for more and messier work.

Raw juices are pure liquid energy. So if blending instead of juicing is the difference between you making your own juice or walking away, give blending a shot.

A Word About Dehydrators

For people interested in going deeper into exploring the raw foods lifestyle, I've included a few recipes in the "Some Like It Raw" Cleanse and Mexican Fiesta chapters (pages 85 and 220, respectively) that require a dehydrator. (There are plenty of recipes that don't require a dehydrator, so you can still do those cleanses without buying one.)

All dehydrators operate basically the same way—heated air is blown over the food until it dries—but it's important to choose one that has an adjustable thermostat. Enzymes degrade at about 118 degrees Fahrenheit, so be mindful of setting the temperature below that. If you get one, other factors to consider are price, the amount of space you have in your kitchen, and total drying area within the dehydrator. Generally, the more drying area, the higher the price.

For home use, I like the Excalibur Small Garden model. It has five trays and a 26-hour timer, but it's the size of a large toaster, so it doesn't take up much counter space. Check online for the best price.

Miscellaneous Other Supplies

Depending on the cleanse you choose, there are other small supplies you might need to make the recipes or do the supportive disciplines, so read the entire chapter beforehand to see what else to pick up in advance.

SEVEN ESSENTIALS OF YOUR DAILY ROUTINE

The seven activities included below are serious cleanse boosters that magnify the positive effects of a cleansing program. They'll ease the physical symptoms you might experience and help you work through the emotions that come up during a cleanse. They'll also help you harness the new levels of energy you'll feel and enhance your clarity, sense of purpose, serenity and balance.

1. Hydrate

Ideally, water makes up 60% to 70% of our body weight. Staying within that range is key to:

* Maintaining endurance and energy levels
* Ensuring that your organs, cells and other internal systems function properly
* Keeping proper muscle and skin tone
* Preventing and relieving constipation

So always drink plenty of water!

This becomes even more important during the detoxification phase of a cleanse. Drinking fluids helps move food through the intestines and flushes the toxins from our blood, organs and cells that get released during the cleansing process.

How much water we need to drink each day differs from one person to another. But as a starting point, I recommend drinking 1 liter of water for each 30 pounds of your body weight during a cleanse (so if you weigh 150 pounds, you should drink 5 liters per day: $150 \div 30 = 5$). That may sound like a lot, but it's vital for any good cleanse. Do the best you can.

While you're cleansing, the following signs could be indications that you're dehydrated and need to increase your intake of water:

* Dark yellow or orange urine

* Dry mouth

* Constipation

* Muscle soreness or cramps

* Joint pain

* Dry skin, poor skin tone or wrinkles

* Swollen legs, feet, hands or face

* Dizziness

* Lethargy or depression

The kind of water you drink is equally important. Pollutants in U.S. tap water, and the chlorine and fluoride added at municipal water treatment plants, increase acidity in the body. So it's best to drink purified water, natural spring water or distilled water—whether you're cleansing or not. (If you don't have a carbon filter installed on your tap at home, I recommend getting one right away.)

NOTE: During meals, limit the amount of liquid you drink to avoid squelching your "digestive fire." If you need a beverage during a meal, I recommend drinking warm lemon water or herbal tea, in moderation.

2. Sweat It Out

One of the most relaxing and effective ways to help flush toxins from the body during a cleanse is doing a steam or a sauna. So grab your swimsuit or a towel and head to your sauna, a local spa or gym for a 10- to 15-minute "sweat session." Make sure not to overdo it. If you feel overheated, get out, take a quick cool shower, and then jump back in. Whether you choose to steam or sauna, don't forget to drink more water to replenish the fluids you sweat out! (Tip: To add an invigorating spin to your sauna, add a few drops of eucalyptus oil to the bucket of water you pour over the lava rocks. It's great for opening up your airways.)

If you'd prefer to sweat it out at home, take a hot bath before going to bed. Remember: the goal is to sweat, so make the water as warm as you can comfortably bear it. Again, if you get overheated, take a quick cool shower or pour some cool water over your head. Boost the cleansing effects of the warm soak by adding a ½ cup of Epsom salts to the bath—they help pull toxins from the body. (Tips: If you're looking for a more sensual soak, add a few drops of lavender or your favorite aromatherapy oil. Or, to really turn up the heat, pour a ½ cup of ginger powder into the tub to elevate your body temperature.)

NOTE: Steams and saunas are not recommended for individuals with high blood pressure or women who are pregnant. Check with your physician to see if you have any other preexisting condition that would preclude you from doing a steam or sauna or taking a hot bath.

3. Move Your Body

Boost the life force flowing through you and get those bowels moving with some daily exercise. The deeper breathing that comes with exercise improves circulation, increases oxygenation in the bloodstream, and helps flush toxins and cellular waste from the body. Moving your body also helps clear your mind—and the endorphins you get from regular exercise are great natural mood enhancers.

Try exercising for at least 30 minutes each day. Your preferred workout is usually best. If you don't have one, go for a brisk walk, run, take a yoga class, head to the gym, dance your feet off, go for a swim, jump on a trampoline, or ride a bike—it's up to you. If you can, get outside and exercise in nature. My personal favorite for getting out of my mind and into my breath and body is a good trail run.

NOTE: Don't start a new, vigorous exercise program during a cleanse.

4. Breathe

The last person who told you to "relax and take a deep breath" was onto something. We tend to take shallow breaths when we're stressed, angry or sad—limiting the amount of life-giving oxygen coming into our bodies and the amount of acidic carbon dioxide leaving our bodies. When we consciously shift out of that state of mind and breathe deeply, the increased oxygen level boosts our metabolism, strengthens our immune system and bolsters cellular functions.

When you start breathing deeply, you can feel your body relaxing, your blood pressure drop and your heart rate slow. You almost instantly feel more calm. Over the longer term, the increased oxygen and decreased carbon dioxide levels that come with deeper breathing have a profound effect on dropping acid levels in the body—and soothing acidic states of mind.

A couple of my favorite breathing exercises follow. Any one of these will help you reap the benefits of deep breathing. As you exhale, visualize impurities, stress and toxins leaving your body. Each time you inhale, imagine the fresh air filling you with energy and purifying your system.

Do them whenever you think about it during the day—particularly if you find yourself stressed out. You'll see they're more than just a breath of fresh air!

The Belly Roll

As you take a slow, deep breath through your nose, imagine the air filling your belly and then your chest. Feel your belly and chest expand with the inhale.

As you exhale completely through your nose, draw in your belly to force out as much air as possible. Pause before slowly inhaling, refilling your belly and then your chest.

Repeat until you feel completely relaxed.

Nadi Sodhana (Alternate-Nostril Breathing)

Yogis believe that alternate-nostril breathing is one of the most effective ways to calm the mind and nervous system, balance the right and left hemispheres of the brain, and clear out channels of energy. While he was teaching a class at my favorite Mill Valley yoga studio, a visiting yogi told us that starting and ending our days with 5 or 10 minutes of nadi sodhana breathing would change our lives. I can't speak for everyone who was there, but I know that I feel much more centered and calm when I devote time to doing this. And I feel like I reap the benefits of an "integrated brain" as well, getting the most out of both my right-brain creative and left-brain analytic juices.

Sit comfortably on the floor or lie down. If you lie down, be sure to maintain the natural curvature of the spine by keeping your cervical and lumbar vertebrae slightly off the floor. You should have enough room to slip your fingers between the floor and your lower back and the floor and your neck. If your lower back is uncomfortable, place a rolled-up towel under your knees.

Close your eyes.

Bring your right hand to your face. With your right thumb, close the right nostril and gently inhale through the left nostril for a count of 4 seconds (don't force the inhale).

At the top of the inhale, use your right ring finger to close your left nostril while removing your thumb from your right nostril. Exhale the breath slowly through the right nostril for 8 seconds.

Then, inhale through the open right nostril for 4 seconds. Close the right nostril with your right thumb, lift your ring finger to open your left nostril, and exhale through the left nostril for 8 seconds. This completes one round of nadi sodhana breathing.

Start with 10 rounds of the breathing and see if you can work your way up to 5 or 10 minutes.

5. Flush Your System

Proper elimination is an important component of the journey toward optimal health, so clearing out the old sludge in your intestines is crucial. When you change your diet, it's not uncommon for your digestion or elimination to change. The effect differs by person and by cleanse, but you may find that things aren't moving properly though the body. If you find you're constipated, there are several options out there to help you stay regular. I suggest that you do either one of the following:

✳ At bedtime, take a natural laxative such as Natural Vitality's Natural Calm (rich in magnesium and calcium), Swiss Kriss or a laxative tea. Products containing pure aloe, aloe leaf, slippery elm, flaxseed, marshmallow root, triphala, yellow dock, and psyllium husks all help move the bowels. They're available at your local health-food stores.

✳ Go the enema or colonic route. If you choose to do the Urban Revitalizer, Winter Wake-Up or Green Buzz cleanses, this step is especially important. Enemas and colonics are the quickest way to remove toxic sludge from the colon, and they also provide fast relief from detox symptoms such as headaches, throbbing joints, constipation and body aches. You can find do-it-yourself formulas at your local health-food store or go to a colon hydrotherapist. Ask your physician or naturopath for a referral if you don't know of a therapist in your area. You can do an enema each day or consult with a colon hydrotherapist about how many colonics to do during a 5- to 7-day cleanse.

NOTE: These remedies are appropriate during a cleanse, but be careful about becoming dependent on them to ensure regularity. On an ongoing basis, a balanced, healthy diet should be what you rely on to avoid constipation.

ERIKA'S THOUGHTS ON COLONICS

When I signed up for one of Adina's cleanses, she recommended I get a colonic. I'd never had one before and wasn't sure that I wanted to. But now that I've done one, I feel like it's a pretty nurturing process. I know that may sound odd, but it was done by a very experienced, calm, and kindly reassuring woman, who explained the process of how we process our food and eliminate—or in some cases, don't eliminate—what we don't need. After the fact, it was amazing just how much detritus from the stresses of life had been tucked into my personal plumbing. It didn't hurt, it wasn't embarrassing—she's a professional and has seen it all—and it was just an hour out of the day. I may not look forward to it the way I would a massage, but it seemed to be an important thing to get my system back in balance. I would say it's necessary to ensure you get the most out of the cleanse, so to speak.

6. Nurture Your Mind and Spirit

Doing meditations is a great way to care for your mind and spirit during a cleanse—even taking just 10 minutes out of your day can have a positive impact. Meditation can help you start your day in a centered, calm state of mind; unplug from stress during the day; and relax as you prepare to sleep.

I've included a meditative exercise in several of the cleansing chapters. You can meditate in silence or with soothing or uplifting music. The goal is to consciously relax your entire body, from head to toe.

As I mentioned earlier, I also recommend keeping a journal. Most people experience greater levels of clarity during a cleanse—so don't be surprised if you experience breakthroughs on issues you've been struggling with. This is also a great time to set intentions for the future. Keep track of your thoughts with an evening journal. Remember to make note of the changes you're seeing and feeling during the cleanse and acknowledge your efforts!

7. Catch Your Zzzzzs

A solid night of sleep is incredibly rejuvenating for the body and spirit. There are several things I recommend doing to put your body and mind into a restful state:

* Avoid exercising, watching intense TV or movies, or read-ing something heavy right before bed.

* Listen to one of your favorite mellow CDs to help you chill out.

* Try consciousness relaxation, breathing exercises or medi-tation to put yourself into a relaxed state and help you sleep more soundly.

﹡ Take a warm bath before bed to help you unplug from the day and prepare for sleep.

If a sound sleep continues to elude you, there are a variety of natural sleep aids available, including chamomile tea, valerian root and calcium-magnesium, to name a few. Ask about the different alternatives at your local health-food store and then check in with your physician to see which natural remedy might be best for you.

THE ONE-DAY WONDER CLEANSE

The One-Day Wonder Cleanse is a lighten-your-body, clear-your-mind cleanse when you throw your hands in the air and say, "Stop the madness!" It's about unplugging and taking care of yourself for a change. You eat light, nutrient-dense, high-enzymatic juices and soups, completely disconnect from your daily routine, and devote an entire day to nothing but loving you! You set the pace and find your own natural rhythm.

Almost all of us need reminders of the importance of balance and the need to set aside time for ourselves on an ongoing basis. So the One-Day Wonder works two ways: First, it's a stepping-stone for people who want to cleanse but are intimidated by the prospect of cleansing for 5 days or making longer-term changes in their eating habits. I want them to see how easy it can be to take that first step, make changes in their diets just once a week, and check in with their bodies to see how they felt when they ate differently and changed their pace. Second, it's a maintenance routine that we can return to once a week to recalibrate our bodies and retrain our brains about what our bodies need to thrive.

Many people jump into a cleanse looking for a quick fix. They want to jump-start weight loss or catapult through some emotional crisis they're facing, but it's a mistake to think that eating well, exercising or meditating for 7 days a year will permanently transform your health. The truth is, an annual or quarterly cleanse can make you look and feel fantastic in the short term, but it isn't a stand-alone solution. We need also to make smart daily choices about what we bring into our bodies and our lives if we want to see lasting change or improvements in our health and get back into balance.

Think about it this way: We take our cars in for regular tune-ups, we check and refill its fluids, we supply the fuel it needs, and we give it a rest if it's been running on overdrive. If we invest in a little ongoing maintenance, the car lasts longer and runs better. Shouldn't we care enough about ourselves to give our body and spirit that same tender loving care?

ABOUT DR. BRIAN CLEMENT

I admire the work of Brian Clement, PhD, LNC, director of the Hippocrates Health Institute in West Palm Beach, Florida. Hippocrates is one of the leaders in the field of natural and complementary health care and education. It was founded on the belief that a pure, enzyme-rich diet, complemented by positive thinking and noninvasive therapies, are essential elements on the path to optimum health. Clement believes a weekly 1-day cleanse, combined with a pure diet and an exercise program, is the best means of self-maintenance at our disposal.

When to Do the Cleanse

If you're new to cleansing and want a gentle entry into the process, try doing this cleanse once a week for a month. You may be surprised at how easy it is and feel ready to try the Laughing Buddha, Three-Day Face-Lift, Karma, or "Some Like It Raw" cleanses. Or maybe you're flying high after doing a longer cleanse and want to build regular tune-ups into your monthly routine. It's also good if you need a periodic, one-day retreat to soothe your soul and care for yourself.

What You'll See and Feel

With the One-Day Wonder, you'll feel a sense of renewal, calm and balance; confidence and pride in taking a day to care for and rejuvenate your body; and a sense that you're worth it!

HOLLY'S TESTIMONIAL

Five years ago, I came back from a trip to Vail feeling really puffy and out of shape. I took a step back and realized that my lifestyle was catching up with me. If I'm not careful, the sheer pace of my life can border on insanity. I do commercial and residential interior design in San Francisco, and my days are booked with back-to-back meetings with clients, architects, installers and vendors. I have to be on all the time, advising clients and coordinating the work of different vendors—there are an infinite number of details to manage.

Growing up, I'd always been an athlete, so I decided enough was enough and began training for triathlons to get fit again. I worked out daily, got enough sleep and tried to take it easy on nights out with friends. After doing a couple of triathlons, I switched gears and got into a boot camp training program that a friend ran (think Marines for female athletes). Over the past 18 months, I've worked up to going several times a week and I feel fantastic—great energy, fit body—and it's become a form of meditation for me. Thoughts of work and the day ahead that start racing through my brain before I even open my eyes in the morning come to a screeching halt as I focus on nothing except what my body's doing in that moment.

As part of my push back to fitness, I also started doing Adina's five-day Winter Wake-Up or Urban Revitalizer cleanses as an annual ritual to clean my body and clear my mind. While I enjoy fine, rich meals now and then, I'd had a fairly good diet up to that point: primarily vegetarian, with fish and the occasional steak thrown in; no caffeine; and almost no gluten or processed sugars. My biggest hurdles, food-wise, were my fondness for chocolate and the nonstop, on-the-go nibbling I'd do during my fast-paced days at work. The cleanses are such great reminders of how fantastic I feel when I eat what's really good for my body, that I wanted to make this more than an annual ritual. I needed to build in periodic "check-in points" with myself where I take time to unplug and relax.

That's where the One-Day Wonder has been incredibly rejuvenating for me. Once or twice a month it gives me the lift and release I need to avoid reaching shut-down phase when I'm balls-to-the-wall over an extended period of time. It's like my own personal decompression chamber that lets me get my body and mind back into equilibrium.

The One-Day Wonder is a day devoted to nothing but me. I feel so free: no phone; no deadlines; no one asking me questions; no place I need to be and no one I need to see. I choose what I need to do for me and take all the time I want doing it. One of my favorite things to do is get out into nature and go for a hike or a run. I practice breathing more deeply as well (in the high-stress environment at work, I catch myself holding my breath sometimes).

I get all my ingredients the night before so there's no part of my day that's lost running errands. I get up, drink my tea and hot lemon water, and crank up the blender. I love the green soup and make it any time I'm craving it—whether I'm doing the One-Day or not.

I recommend the One-Day Wonder as a great way to get the body and mind back in check.

CLEANSE AT A GLANCE

On waking: Hot Lemon Water

Breakfast: Easy Smoothie

Lunch: Sassy Sausalito Salad with Lemony Quinoa

Snack: Watermelon Salad

Dinner: Blissful Blend Soup

Special Equipment

✳ High-speed blender

RECIPES

LEMON WATER

Makes 1 serving

Lemon water does more than hydrate the body: It also dissolves mucus, flushes the liver, improves the absorption of minerals, encourages the formation of bile (which is critical to digestion) and breaks down fat. So drink it throughout the day! Start with a hot cup in the morning, but then feel free to enjoy it warm or at room temperature all day long. Drinking iced beverages cools the digestive fires, so avoid cold drinks!

16 ounces purified water
2 tablespoons fresh-squeezed lemon juice
Optional: pinch of cayenne pepper

Directions: Stir lemon juice and optional cayenne into water. Pour into a glass and enjoy. To drink this beverage hot, boil the water before adding the lemon juice.

EASY SMOOTHIE

Makes 1 serving

This smoothie is a quick pick-me-up that's sure to get you started on the right foot. The added protein powder sustains you through the morning. Be sure to choose a non-whey, non-soy-based protein powder—I love Vega's Whole Food Health Optimizer.

1 cup unsweetened almond milk
1 cup water
2 scoops protein powder
½ cup berries of your choice

Directions: Add all ingredients to a blender and process until smooth.

SASSY SAUSALITO SALAD
WITH LEMONY QUINOA

Makes 1 serving

This is one of my favorite salads. The combination of the crunchy cabbage, the creamy avocado and the tangy quinoa makes for a taste sensation!

Salad
½ head romaine lettuce, chopped into bite-sized pieces
½ cup shredded cabbage

½ cup arugula or spinach
½ avocado, peeled, seeded and chopped into ½-inch dice
1 tablespoon raw almonds or toasted sesame seeds

Directions: Mix the romaine, cabbage, arugula and avocado together in a large bowl. Chop the almonds. Pour the lemony quinoa and dressing over salad and toss well. Transfer to a plate or eat it right out of the bowl!

LEMONY QUINOA

½ cup water
¼ cup quinoa, rinsed and drained
2 tablespoons chopped cilantro
1 tablespoon fresh lemon juice

Directions: Boil the water in a small saucepan. Add the quinoa and cover. Cook over low heat for 12 minutes, until al dente. Transfer to a bowl and toss with cilantro and lemon juice.

DRESSING

2 tablespoons flax or olive oil
1 lemon, juiced
¼ teaspoon garlic, minced
Pinch of Himalayan or Celtic sea salt

Directions: Whisk together the flax or olive oil, lemon juice, garlic, and salt in a small bowl.

WATERMELON SALAD

Makes 2 servings

This salad is an excellent source of vitamins C and A and beta-carotene. Watermelon is refreshing and hydrating, and its pink color is a sign that it is also packed with the potent carotenoid antioxidant lycopene. This powerful antioxidant travels through the body, neutralizing free radicals. You could choose to eat the watermelon alone, but the additional ingredients add more nutrients, bulk and contrasting flavors.

Salad

2 cups watermelon, cut into bite-sized cubes after the rind
   has been removed
2 cups arugula, julienned
¼ cup jicama, peeled and chopped into small dice
1 tablespoon raw pumpkinseeds, soaked overnight

Directions: Add all ingredients to a medium bowl with dressing and toss to combine.

ZIPPY LIME DRESSING

2 tablespoons flax or olive oil
1 teaspoon fresh lime juice
Pinch of Himalayan or Celtic sea salt

Directions: Whisk all ingredients together in a small bowl.

BLISSFUL BLEND SOUP

1 serving

This raw soup is a powerful blend. It helps stimulate the immune system and has antibacterial and antifungal properties. All the nutrients are delivered blended, so it's easy to digest—and tastes delicious, too.

2 cups spinach, chopped
1½ cup water
1 small avocado, pitted, peeled, and chopped
2 tablespoons fresh lemon juice
1 teaspoon minced yellow onion
⅛ teaspoon Himalayan or Celtic sea salt
Hot sauce or chili paste to taste (I load it up!)

Directions: Blend all ingredients in blender at high speed for five seconds.

Cleanse-Boosting Activities

Make It a One-Day Retreat
You're giving yourself the gift of recalibrating your system, so why not make it a more holistic healing experience by checking out of the daily grind and checking into yourself? Take a day off work, or do this over a weekend when you have no plans. Unplug the phone, turn off the television, let your friends know you're going undercover for the day, and think about what it is you really want to do to unwind. Maybe you'll pick up that book you've been wanting to read or draw yourself a hot bath or go on a scenic ride or hit that hiking trail you've been meaning to explore—whatever feels like bliss to you!

Think Positive!

Kick the day off with the following affirmations:

I have the power to make changes in my body, my attitude and my life.

I am self-motivated—I decide what to put into my body.

I am self-generating—my thoughts and habits shape my body.

Brush It Off

The skin is the largest organ in our body and is responsible for about 25% of our detoxification daily, so give your skin a helping hand. Shed dead skin cells, stimulate the circulatory and lymphatic systems, and eliminate toxins from the body by dry-brushing your body before showering or bathing. First, buy a brush: any long-handled, natural-bristle brush will do the job. Then, before you bathe, simply stand in the shower or tub and—starting with your feet—use circular motions to brush your limbs and torso in the direction of your heart. Bathe or shower after brushing.

Bathe Balinese Style

This sensual bath will titillate your senses of smell, touch and taste. Close your eyes and escape to the islands! The young coconuts and tinctures are available at health-food stores.

Bath filled with hot water
2 young coconuts
3 drops ginger tincture
3 drops orange tincture
1 straw
Candles and music of your choice

Directions: Draw a bath of hot water. While the bath is filling, open the two coconuts (see directions on page 160). Light the candles and put on your favorite relaxing music—I like Indonesian tunes to really transport me to Bali. Add the coconut water from one coconut and the ginger and orange tinctures to the bathwater. Get into the bath, pop the straw into the second coconut, and sip while you soak! Ahhh . . .

When you're through with your bath, rub coconut oil into your body and then take a quick, cool shower to stimulate your circulatory and lymph systems.

THE LAUGHING BUDDHA CLEANSE (5 DAYS)

I f you haven't ever thought much about what you consume day to day and want a soft entry into the world of eating well, the Laughing Buddha Cleanse may be just the place to start. The dishes are flavorful and satisfying, which might help you stick with the program for the full 5 days and open the door to making lasting changes to your diet in the future.

Why Buddha? Because his name translates to "the one who woke up," and this vegetarian detox diet is a gentle wake-up to the power of food as medicine. I picked the Laughing Buddha because this cleanse is a joyful celebration of the bountiful life you can have when you're free of the foods that muddle your mind and create dis-ease in the body. In combination with the meditation exercises (part of Buddha's own path to enlightenment), it can transform the way you feel and look at life. If you've lived life at a pace that hasn't allowed time to experience the rejuvenation of sitting quietly and enjoying the present moment, this cleanse can be an emotional and spiritual awakening as well.

HOLD THE MEAT, PLEASE

Famous vegetarians throughout history, including Mahatma Gandhi, Mawlana Jala ad-Din Muhammad Rumi, Sir Isaac Newton, Coretta Scott King, Albert Einstein, Jane Goodall, Charles Darwin, Leonardo da Vinci, Vincent van Gogh, Louisa May Alcott, Bob Marley and Joan Baez, understood that trying to digest meats saps vital creative and spiritual energy. A vegetarian diet brings greater clarity, a higher level of consciousness and productivity, and a deeper connection to the divine.

Get ready to be pleasantly surprised at how delicious vegetarian cuisine can be. It won't take you long to see that eating a balanced vegetarian diet can heal your body and make you feel great too.

Got Zen?

Often, we get so busy planning our next steps that we miss the moment we're in. Zen Buddhism teaches us to still our minds. When we get into a calm, relaxed state, focusing on the present, ideas or guidance we've needed can come to us without our actively searching or pushing for them. That's what being in the moment is all about: becoming still, opening up to the flow and allowing the answers to come.

There's a passage in the book *Being Peace*, by Thich Nhat Hanh, that captures this so well. Hanh says, "We do so much, we run so quickly, the situation is so difficult, and many people say, 'Don't just sit there, do something.' But doing more things may make the situation worse. So, you should say, 'Don't just do something, sit there.' Sit there, stop, be yourself first, and begin from there. That's the meaning of meditation."

As you'll see, each of the cleansing chapters in this book includes a different form of meditation, because, in my opinion, there's no one "right way" to meditate. You can sit quietly in silence, take a walk on a beach listening to the surf, ride a bike, dance or take a run—whatever clears your mind and keeps you in the present moment. I focus on Zen meditation in this chapter because it was the first form of meditation I learned, and I was creating and eating many of the recipes included in this cleanse while I was practicing it.

As a society, we have so much resistance around being still and present in the moment. We're not wired that way—we're bombarded with stimuli, and our minds are used to chasing different thoughts at every turn. So start meditating in small doses. If you can't escape your thoughts at first, try not to get frustrated. The key here is to keep setting aside a time and place to turn the mind off and just be. Enlightenment is no easy job, so keep a sense of humor and be kind to yourself. Let the Laughing Buddha be a reminder: If meditation gets derailed by different thoughts, don't get upset; just laugh and start again. It's not about how good you are, it's about sticking with it—that's why it's called a "practice!" Let go of the past and the future and rediscover the serenity and beauty that can be found in the here and now. That's what the Laughing Buddha cleanse is all about!

When to Do the Cleanse

Do the Laughing Buddha Cleanse if the food you're eating leaves you feeling sluggish and lethargic; if you want to make dietary changes but need a gentle start to make them stick; if you've been thinking about experimenting with vegetarian food and want a healthy, balanced way to start; if you're looking to spark creative and physical energy; if you'd like to awaken your heart or restore a sense of peace and a connection to the divine in your life; if you're starving for deeper nourishment.

This cleanse is gentle enough to do up to once a month.

What You'll See and Feel

During the cleanse, you'll feel lighter and experience a boost in energy. Your skin tone and coloring will improve, and you may lose weight. You'll have greater mental clarity and emotional balance. You'll awaken your sense of spirit and realize you're connected to everything and everyone around you.

DOROTHY'S TESTIMONIAL

Since I was 14 years old, I've varied between widely different diets. I experimented with being vegetarian and vegan, and then reintroduced chicken as a meat source (a fad diet dubbed the California Vegetarian). Then, from the ages of 24 through 34, I pretty much fell off the wagon. I was always on the run, eating horrible processed and fast foods. Anything that was quick and tasty was fair game, and I'd try to make myself feel better by saying it was "just a treat."

I'd always loved cooking but tended to make rich and fattening "indulgence" foods that satisfied my desire to cook more than my body's holistic needs. As a result, I was unable to maintain a consistent weight and healthy constitution. Then it all came to a head when I was diagnosed with serious thyroid problems and had to have my thyroid removed. Once I recovered, I immediately took a look at my overall lifestyle and decided to make changes in my diet—it was the area where I was in the most dire need of help, and I thought my passion for cooking would help me get through it.

The first thing I had to do was figure out what I should eat that would nurture my body and improve my health. So in 2006, I applied to Bauman College in Berkeley, California, a holistic nutrition and culinary arts school devoted to using whole, organic, vegetarian foods to restore metabolic balance in the body. I learned to create a diet that meets my specific needs and supports local farmers and sustainable organic agriculture.

As I began replacing the bad foods in my diet and purged toxic food and waste from my body, I was amazed to see how whole foods could be such a source of healing. I felt grounded, but I had this vibrant energy. My absorption of the thyroid replacement hormone improved so much after switching to whole foods that my dosage was cut far sooner than my doctors had thought would be possible. The better the foods I cooked, the better I felt!

In addition to eating whole, vegan foods, I made a concerted effort to slow down. I did 3-minute meditations throughout the day to recalibrate my state of mind. (In the early days they were crucial in helping me avoid the temptation of comfort foods too.) Rather than eating on the go in the car, I made mealtimes a ritual where I ate more slowly and chewed more thoroughly. Together, these things helped my body assimilate nutrients instead of stressing it.

I was lucky not to experience the typical detox symptoms someone might have when switching from a "standard American diet" to whole foods, because I started gently. I replaced one bad thing a week with something better, so the crossover was gradual and remarkably kind.

Learning how the wrong foods can cause adverse reactions has helped me get more in tune with my body and develop a healthier relationship with food. With my newfound knowledge I've been able to create exciting foods that my family and friends love. Chef Adina was one of my instructors at Bauman, and she played a big part in cultivating my awareness of the incredible benefits of holistic eating. I still use and recommend the personal techniques she shared with me in our classes! To this day, I do vegetarian cleanses once a month to recalibrate my system.

Today, I'm a purchasing chef at a restaurant, working with the executive chef to create menus that utilize the local bounty of organic whole foods. And I'm still struck by how satisfying meals outside the whole meat-starch-veggie structure can be. A combination of grains, legumes, greens, seeds, teas, juices, superfoods, vegetables and fruits are amazingly satiating. And knowing that I'm eating a diet in harmony with the Earth affects all aspects of my life—how I feel, how I interact with others, and the impact I have on my community. I can't recommend a vegetarian cleanse enough!

THE MISSING INGREDIENT

Good, clean food prepared with love tastes better and is more nourishing. We're so rushed, it's easy to overlook that simple, powerful ingredient. Fresh food is alive and takes on our energy and moods, so it's affected by the manner in which we prepare it. Keep that in mind when you follow the recipes I've shared with you. Food cooked by an unhappy or stressed-out chef isn't good for your health!

CLEANSE AT A GLANCE

On waking: Hot Lemon Water (see recipe on page 33)

Breakfast: Selection from the breakfast options

Snack, if needed: 1 serving Chia-Citrus Drink or Buddha's Mint Lemonade

Lunch: Selection from the lunch options

Snack, if needed: Tea and ½ an apple, small cucumber or bell pepper, or 1 medium carrot

Dinner: Selection from the dinner options

Special Equipment

* Juicer

* High-speed blender

* Nut-milk bag (available at health-food stores)

* Fine sieve

RECIPES

NOTE: Ingredients such as raw agave syrup, stevia, chia seeds, MSM (methylsulfonylmethane), green powder, nori sheets, brown-rice vinegar, umeboshi vinegar, chickpea miso, kombu, raw sauerkraut and young coconuts are available at health-food stores. Wheatgrass shots can be purchased at juice bars or health-food stores.

Green powder is a blend of cereal grasses, vegetables and algae. Vitamineral Green, Green Magic and Dr. Robert Young's pH Miracle greens are three green powders I recommend.

Breakfast Choices

GREEN GANDHI*

Makes one 16-ounce serving

The kale, lemon, and apple in this recipe are a great liver-cleansing combination, and the juice is delicious too!

1 head romaine lettuce
5 kale leaves
½-inch piece of fresh ginger
1 medium cucumber
Optional: ½ a pear, cored
½ lemon, juiced
Purified water as needed

---

* Denotes recipes that are appropriate for breaking the stringent cleanses—the Urban Revitalizer, Winter Wake-Up and Green Buzz.

Directions: Cut the first four ingredients and the pear, if you choose to add it, into pieces small enough to fit into the feeder tube of your juicer, and juice. Start with the romaine and end with the cucumber to be sure to get all the juice out of the kale. Pour juice into a glass. Add the optional green powder, lemon juice and enough water to make a 16-ounce serving. Stir and enjoy.

ORANGE SMOOTHIE*

Makes 1 serving

This recipe calls for oranges, but you can experiment with different fruits. I sometimes use mango or papaya.

3 juicing oranges, peeled and pulled apart into sections
1 cup ice
1 teaspoon minced gingerroot

Directions: Toss all ingredients into a blender and process until smooth. Pour into a glass and enjoy!

GOLDILOCKS'S APPLE–BERRY PORRIDGE

Makes 2 servings

This recipe is packed with fiber to keep digestion rolling along, and the apple-pumpkin combination gives it a great texture. The flax-seed adds crunch and ensures that you get your daily dose of healthy omega-3 fatty acids.

1 large apple, peeled, cored and chopped into large dice
1 cup berries of your choice

¼ cup pumpkinseeds, soaked overnight
Pinch of Himalayan or Celtic sea salt
Optional: 2 dried figs, cut in half
Garnish: 1 tablespoon flaxseed, ground in a spice mill or well-cleaned
    coffee grinder

Directions: Blend the first four ingredients and the figs, if you want to use them, in a food processor until smooth. Pour mixture into a bowl and sprinkle with ground flaxseed. Enjoy!

RISE-UP MILLET

Makes 4 servings

Enjoy this cold or hot—whatever feels more satisfying to you. To get a change of flavors, you can substitute 1 cup quinoa for the millet, but be sure to add ¼ cup of water to the recipe.

1¾ cups purified water
1 cup millet, rinsed well in a fine sieve
1 cup almond milk (if you'd like to make your own almond milk, follow
    the recipe on page 93)
4 teaspoons unsweetened coconut flakes
Agave syrup or stevia to taste
4 teaspoons chopped almonds, walnuts, macadamia nuts or raw
    pumpkinseeds

Directions: After rinsing the millet, toast it in a saucepan over medium-high heat until fragrant and lightly colored. In a separate pot, bring water to a boil and add the millet. Reduce to simmer and cook for 15 minutes or until all water is absorbed, stirring periodically. Remove from heat and let stand for 10 minutes, covered. At this stage, the millet will keep for several days, refrigerated in a sealed container.

For each serving, put a ½ cup millet into a cereal bowl and add ¼ cup almond milk, 1 teaspoon coconut flakes, the agave syrup or stevia, and 1 teaspoon of your choice of nut or pumpkinseeds. Stir and enjoy. If you're using previously prepared and refrigerated millet, warm gently on the stove until just heated, prior to serving.

"HELLO, WORLD!" SMOOTHIE

Makes one 16-ounce serving

This smoothie is packed with nutrients that get your day off to a great start: MSM (methylsulfonylmethane) is a naturally occurring sulfur compound that's great for skin, hair and nails. Note: If you're allergic to bee stings, omit the raw honey.

2 cups purified water
¼ cup hemp seeds
5 dried figs, soaked for 1 hour to rehydrate
⅛ teaspoon MSM (1 capsule, opened)
Pinch of stevia or 2 teaspoons raw honey
Pinch of Himalayan or Celtic sea salt

Directions: Add all ingredients to your blender and process until smooth. Pour into a glass and enjoy.

Lunch Choices

NOTE: If you'd like a protein or enzymatic boost, add sprouts to any of the lunch or dinner recipes. My favorites are sunflower, pea and mung bean.

BIG OL' CHOPPED SALAD*

Makes 2 servings

For this salad, you can use any vegetable you love, chopped into small dice. Save time by making a couple of servings at a time so you can snack on it for a couple of days. The Lemon Terrific Tahini Dressing is light and adds a bit of zip to the veggie combination—it's also a yummy dressing for steamed veggies and a makes a great dip.

Salad

1 medium tomato
1 avocado, peeled and pitted
1 endive
1 cup cabbage, shredded
1 small zucchini
1 medium beet, peeled and cut into small pieces
1 cup baby arugula
1 cup romaine leaves
1/2 fennel bulb
1/2 cup sugar snap peas
5 olives of your choice, pitted and chopped
Optional garnish: pine nuts or raw sauerkraut

Directions: Chop all ingredients into small dice. Transfer to a large bowl and toss. Store half the salad for another meal. Add half the dressing to the remaining salad and toss. Sprinkle on optional pine nuts or sauerkraut to add protein to the meal.

LEMON TERRIFIC TAHINI DRESSING

1/2 cup raw tahini
3 tablespoons purified water
1/3 cup fresh lime, lemon or grapefruit juice

½ cucumber, peeled
½ clove garlic, minced

Directions: Put all ingredients into your blender and blend until smooth. If needed, add small amount of water to thin the dressing. Dressing can be stored in your refrigerator in a sealed container for up to 1 week.

JICAMA SALAD*

Makes 1 serving

On a hot summer day, this is a really refreshing salad. The crunch of the jicama, the cool creaminess of the avocado and the zip of the vinaigrette are a great combo.

Salad
1 small jicama, peeled and julienned
Juice of 1 lime
Pinch of Himalayan or Celtic sea salt
2 tablespoons raw pumpkinseeds
1 avocado, pitted, peeled and chopped into ½-inch dice

Directions: Toss first four ingredients together in a bowl. Fold in avocado and 2 tablespoons of the citrus vinaigrette.

CITRUS VINAIGRETTE

½ cup olive or flax oil
½ cup fresh lime or lemon juice
Pinch of Himalayan or Celtic sea salt
Pinch of black pepper

Directions: Whisk ingredients together until blended.

GREEN SPLIT-PEA SOUP

Makes 4 servings

This is a deliciously healthy twist on traditional split-pea soup: The miso has a lovely nutty flavor and the kombu adds vital sea minerals to the soup.

4½ cups purified water
1 cup green split peas, rinsed several times
1 small strip kombu seaweed
1 teaspoon ginger, peeled and finely minced
1 clove garlic, minced
1 onion, chopped
1 medium carrot, chopped into small dice
1 stalk celery, chopped into small dice
1 tablespoon chickpea miso
1 teaspoon umeboshi vinegar
1 shiso leaf, finely julienned

Directions: Bring water to boil in a 3-quart pot. Add peas and continue boiling on medium-high heat until peas are soft, skimming foam and adding more water as needed. Add kombu, ginger, garlic, and onion and simmer for 30 minutes, covered. Add the carrot and celery and simmer for 30 minutes more. Remove from heat and discard the kombu. Stir in the miso and vinegar. Ladle into serving bowl and garnish with shiso leaf.

GREEN VEGGIES À LA ADINA*

Makes 2 servings

This hands-down crowd-pleaser is the signature dish that I bring to holiday parties and dinner parties. The lemon juice and olives add a tang that makes this dish pop.

1 cup broccoli, chopped
1 large handful of green beans
2 tablespoons olive oil
3 tablespoons fresh lemon juice
⅛ teaspoon Himalayan or Celtic sea salt
2 tablespoons Moroccan olives, pitted and chopped

Directions: Blanch broccoli and green beans in boiling water with 1 teaspoon salt until crisp tender, 5 to 8 minutes. Meanwhile, whisk together the oil, lemon juice and salt in a medium bowl. When veggies are done, transfer them to a bowl with the dressing and toss. Transfer the veggies to a plate, garnish with olives and serve.

MARJORAM RICE

Makes 4 servings

I love making this dish for my friends. The flavors blend together magically and we have fun eating it rolled up in steamed cabbage leaves. The Lemon Terrific Tahini Dressing (page 50) is great on this.

2 cups purified water
2 tablespoons olive oil
Pinch of salt
1 cup brown rice
2 tablespoons marjoram, chopped
2 tablespoons fresh lemon juice
½ teaspoon Himalayan or Celtic sea salt
½ cup raw pine nuts or raw mung bean sprouts (see page 149 for sprouting instructions)

Directions: In a 2-quart saucepan, bring the water, 1 tablespoon oil and the salt to a boil. Stir in rice. Lower heat and simmer rice, covered, for 45 minutes, until it's cooked through and the water has evaporated. Remove from heat and let rest for 5 minutes. Add the second tablespoon of oil and the remaining ingredients and stir. Transfer one portion to a bowl and enjoy.

QUINOA WITH PÂTÉ À LA SHAMAH

Makes 4 servings

This dish knocks it out of the park. In addition to being chock-full of nutrients, quinoa is gluten-free and easily digested and acts as a "prebiotic," feeding healthy bacteria in your intestines. Quinoa is an ancient grainlike seed grown in Peru. It's a nutritional powerhouse that has more amino acids, enzymes, vitamins, minerals, fiber, antioxidants, and phytonutrients than most grains, so you get all those nutrients without totally "carbing up." You can enjoy this alone or with a salad or steamed veggies.

Pâté à la Shamah

1 cup raw almonds
½ cup hemp seeds
1 cup arugula
1 cup cilantro, chopped
1 clove garlic, minced
3 tablespoons lemon juice
1 red or yellow pepper, chopped into large dice
Pinch of Himalayan or Celtic sea salt

Directions: Put all ingredients into a food processor and blend until the mixture is the consistency of pesto. Transfer it to bowl or airtight container for future use. The pâté will keep, refrigerated, for up to 3 days.

QUINOA

---

1 cup quinoa, rinsed several times
1¾ cups purified water
2 tablespoons fresh lemon juice
⅓ cup cilantro, chopped
1 green onion, chopped
2 tablespoons olive oil
Pinch of Himalayan or Celtic sea salt

Directions: Add quinoa to boiling water. When it returns to a boil, lower to simmer and cover. Cook until water is absorbed, about 15 to 20 minutes. Remove from heat and let stand, covered, for 10 minutes. Transfer the quinoa to a separate bowl and toss with cilantro, green onion, olive oil, salt and pepper. Mix in 3 or more tablespoons of the Pâté à la Shamah. Transfer to a bowl and serve.

ISRAELI CHOPPED SALAD*

Makes 1 serving

When I was growing up, my mother always had a fresh container of this salad in our fridge. I love the combination of flavors.

1 cup cucumber, chopped into small dice
1 cup tomato, chopped
4 tablespoons parsley, chopped
1 tablespoon Kalamata or Moroccan olives, pitted and chopped
Pinch of Himalayan or Celtic sea salt
Pinch of black pepper

Directions: Add all ingredients to a medium bowl and toss them. Transfer the salad to a plate and serve.

Snack Choices

CHIA–CITRUS DRINK

Makes 1 serving

This recipe was inspired by Dorothy Kinney, one of my students at Bauman College in Berkeley, California. Chia seeds were staples of the pre-Columbian Aztecs, Mayans and Indians of the U.S. Southwest. They're a source of complete proteins and essential fatty acids and are packed with calcium and antioxidants. The chemical properties of chia also aid the absorption of nutrients. Altogether, it's an ancient superfood and a really filling snack too.

Chia-Citrus Drink
1 tablespoon chia gel
1 cup purified water
1 cup unsweetened citrus juice of your choice

Directions: Add the chia gel, citrus juice and water to a glass and enjoy.

CHIA GEL

1 tablespoon chia seeds
1 cup purified water

Directions: The evening before you plan to make the citrus drink, add dry chia seeds to water in a covered mason jar and shake the jar. After 15 minutes, shake it again to disperse any clumps, and then leave it in refrigerator overnight. Chia gel will last for 2 weeks in the refrigerator.

BUDDHA'S MINT LEMONADE

Makes 1 serving

The mountains in Park City, Utah, gave me the inspiration for this refreshing cooler. Talk about your natural highs!

2 cups purified water
1 herbal mint tea bag
Juice of 1 lemon
2 teaspoons agave syrup or pinch of stevia

Directions: Bring water to a boil on the stove. Remove from heat, add teabag, and steep for 5 minutes. Stir in lemon juice and agave or stevia. Chill until cool or drink warm.

Dinner Choices

BLANCHED GREENS WITH SPICY ASIAN DRESSING*

Makes 1 serving

I never thought that I would crave blanched greens, but then I ate them with this dressing. Its sweet spiciness softens the bitterness of the greens. I make this with kale, collard greens, beet greens, arugula, chard or bok choy.

Greens
3 cups leafy greens of your choice
1 teaspoon Himalayan or Celtic sea salt

Directions: Put 3 quarts of water into a 5-quart pot and bring to a boil. Add salt. Add leafy greens, blanching them for 2 minutes.

Strain them immediately, pushing out the excess water with a spoon. Add 2 to 3 tablespoons of the Asian dressing, transfer to a bowl, and serve.

ASIAN DRESSING

This sauce is also great as a dipping sauce for the sushi or poured over your favorite steamed vegetables. Shoyu is an unpasteurized soy sauce that's available at health-food stores.

1 teaspoon shoyu
1 teaspoon brown rice vinegar
1/2 teaspoon sesame oil
1/2 teaspoon ginger, peeled and finely minced

Directions: Whisk all ingredients together in a small bowl. Pour over blanched greens and serve.

MEXICAN LENTIL STEW

Makes 4 servings

Lentils are a great source of protein and fiber, and this soup is dynamite and flavorful and lasts for a week in your fridge. Enjoy it with a serving of salad for dinner.

1 tablespoon olive oil
1 large yellow or red onion, chopped into medium dice
1 small carrot, chopped into medium dice
2 celery stalks, chopped into medium dice
1/2 teaspoon jalapeño, minced
1/8 teaspoon cumin
1 bay leaf

¼ teaspoon chili powder

3 cloves garlic, minced

One 15-ounce can organic diced tomatoes (get fire-roasted tomatoes
   if you can)

5 cups purified water

1 teaspoon Himalayan or Celtic sea salt

1 cup red or yellow lentils, rinsed well and picked over to remove any
   rocks

One 15-ounce can of organic artichoke hearts, drained and sliced

1 teaspoon cilantro, chopped

Optional garnishes: diced red onion and diced avocado

Directions: Heat oil in a heavy pot. Add onions, carrots, celery, jalapeño, cumin, bay leaf, chili powder and garlic and sauté until onions are translucent. Add tomatoes, water, salt and lentils. Bring to a gentle boil and then simmer for 30 minutes. Add artichoke hearts and cook for another 20 minutes. Remove from heat and stir in cilantro. Ladle into a bowl, garnish with optional red onion and avocado, and serve.

SUSHI ROLLS WITH UME DIPPING SAUCE

Makes 2 servings

The orange juice and umeboshi vinegar marry nicely to make a great alternative dipping sauce for folks allergic to soy. Even if you like soy sauce, you may never go back! To make rolling the sushi easier, you can pick up a sushi mat in Asian markets.

Sushi Rolls

2 cups cooked short-grain brown rice

4 tablespoons brown-rice vinegar

4 nori sheets
3 tablespoons toasted sesame seeds
1 cucumber, cut into 3-inch julienne strips
1 avocado, peeled, pitted and julienned
1 medium yam, baked, peeled and cut into thin slices

Directions: Mix together the rice and vinegar in a bowl. Place 1 nori sheet, shiny side down, on a sushi mat or cutting board. Spread ½ cup rice over nori sheet, leaving ½-inch border along edges. Sprinkle ½ teaspoon sesame seeds over the rice. Place strips of cucumber, avocado and yam at bottom edge of the nori sheet. Roll the nori sheet into a tight cylinder, starting from a short end. Repeat with remaining ingredients. Chill up to 3 hours. Slice rolls into 6 or 7 pieces with sharp knife. Serve with dipping sauce.

UME DIPPING SAUCE

¼ cup umeboshi vinegar
4 tablespoons fresh orange juice
1 scallion, white part only, finely chopped

Directions: Put all ingredients into a small bowl and whisk together.

CURRIED SQUASH SOUP*

Makes 6 servings

The trick to preparing this soup quickly is to cut the vegetables into small pieces or as thinly as possible. Don't be intimidated by the unusual shape and tough skin of butternut squash. It peels easily with a swivel peeler or sharp serrated knife. If unavailable, substitute with peeled sweet potatoes.

5 cups vegetable broth
1 tablespoon olive oil
2 cloves garlic, minced
1½ cups celery, chopped into small dice
1 cup onion, chopped into small dice
½ cup carrot, chopped into small dice
1 tablespoon curry powder
1 tablespoon fresh ginger, minced
½ teaspoon plus pinch of Himalayan or Celtic sea salt
5 cups butternut squash or kabocha squash, peeled and thinly sliced
    into 2-inch pieces
1 teaspoon apple cider or umeboshi vinegar
Optional garnish: toasted pumpkinseeds and dash of cayenne

Directions: In small saucepan, bring 3 cups broth to a boil over high heat. Meanwhile, in large, heavy saucepan, heat oil over medium heat. Add garlic, celery, onion, carrot, curry powder, ginger, and pinch of salt and cook, stirring often, for 5 minutes. Increase heat to high and stir in boiling broth, squash and remaining ½ teaspoon salt. Bring to a boil, cover, reduce heat to medium and cook 10 minutes. Uncover saucepan and stir well with wooden spoon until squash breaks down easily. Remove from heat and stir in apple cider or umeboshi vinegar. Transfer mixture, in batches, to a blender and blend until smooth. Ladle a serving into a bowl, garnish with optional pumpkinseeds and cayenne, and serve.

FEZ-WORTHY FALAFEL

Makes 4 servings

I love this nonfried version of falafel. It tastes excellent and is much healthier than its deep-fried cousin that you get at a falafel stand.

1 cup cooked chickpeas (also called garbanzo beans)
3 teaspoons cooked short-grain rice
1 tablespoon fresh lemon juice
4 tablespoons raw macadamia nuts, chopped
2 tablespoons parsley, minced
1/2 small cucumber, peeled and diced
1/8 teaspoon cumin powder
1 tablespoon fresh lemon juice
Lettuce leaves of your choice

Place all ingredients into a food processor and blend until well mixed. Shape mixture into 1-inch balls. Put 2 balls into a lettuce leaf. If you'd like, add a few spoonfuls of the Israeli Chopped Salad (page 55) and some Lemon Terrific Tahini Dressing (page 50) or a couple of spoonfuls of Great Guac (page 110). Put on a plate and dig in!

MARVELOUS MISO SOUP*

Makes 2 servings

Miso soup is light, yet it's really filling as well. I find it helps me get grounded after a long day at work. The optional ingredients in this recipe add a yummy twist to the broth.

3 cups purified water
1 green onion, thinly chopped
1 clove garlic, minced
1 teaspoon fresh ginger, peeled and minced
Pinch of mustard powder
2 tablespoons chickpea or barley miso (also called red miso)
1/2 teaspoon sesame oil
Squeeze of fresh lemon juice

Optional: handful of sprouts of your choice, 2 tablespoons chopped
  tomato, 2 tablespoons chopped avocado

Directions: Bring the water to a boil in a medium saucepan. Reduce heat and stir in the green onion, ginger, garlic and mustard powder. Cover and simmer for 10 minutes. Remove from heat, add miso paste, and stir until dissolved. Add the sesame oil, lemon juice and optional ingredients of your choice. Ladle a serving into a bowl and enjoy.

TASTE-OF-THE-MED SOUP

Makes 1 serving

This raw soup is energizing and light as a meal or snack on a hot day. *Opa!*

1 cucumber, peeled and cut into large dice
½ apple, cored, peeled and cut into large dice
2 cups arugula, julienned
1 medium avocado, peeled and pitted
1 tablespoon lemon juice
1 cup purified water
½ cup sprouts
1 tablespoon fresh mint, minced, or more to taste
½ teaspoon oregano
Pinch of Himalayan or Celtic sea salt

Directions: Put all ingredients into a blender and pulse until blended, but still a bit chunky. Ladle into a bowl and serve.

Cleanse-Boosting Activities

Go Retro Zen

In this activity, we pay homage to that '70s fad, pet rocks. Hey, it's the Laughing Buddha Cleanse, so stick with me for a minute and play along! First, find a rock you like—any shape will do, but you want it to be large enough for you to write a word on. Next, write down words that are meaningful to you on a piece of paper. Some suggestions: *rebirth, inspiration, life, abundance, peace, prosperity, giving, love, friendship, growth, patience, kindness, beauty, gifts, flow, courage, presence, strength, acceptance, gratitude, serenity, clarity, compassion, gentleness.* From your list, pick the word that speaks to you most right now and paint or write it on your rock; you can make it subtle with just the word, or go to town decorating the entire rock. Go where the spirit takes you. Once you're done, place your rock somewhere where you'll see it at the start and end of your day. Each time it catches your eye, take a minute to unplug, pause, and reflect on your word and what its message can be (or has been) in your life that day. It might sound corny, but you'll be surprised how shifting mental gears into neutral for even a couple of minutes can give you a fresh perspective on the day. Make some for your friends and quietly leave them around their homes or apartments if you want to spread the Zen!

Free Your Mind (and the Rest Will Follow)

Take time each day to sit in grateful meditation. If you're a meditation veteran and have your own routine, good for you! You may prefer your own practice, but here's a meditative exercise that brings me great joy. I do it at sunrise to start my day fully present and aware:

＊ Sit in a comfortable, peaceful place. It can be anywhere—inside or out—where you won't be interrupted.

* Close your eyes. Listen to and feel the inhalation and exhalation of each breath.

* Try to keep your mind from wandering one step into the future or back into the past. Be here now, focused on your breath. This Zen practice of being present in the moment is much like "the art of allowing," where we sit still and allow the universe to bring us messages we need to hear. You're not trying to make something happen; you're simply in a place where you can be open to receiving divine guidance.

* If thoughts continue running through your mind, say, "Be fully present" or "Thinking." Go easy on yourself: These thoughts aren't bad! Smile and go back to focusing on your breath, without frustration or judgment.

* If you still find it difficult to unplug from your thoughts, try this mantra, which is a favorite of my friend Alan Olson, original founder of the San Francisco tall-ship sailing program Call of the Sea, who's been practicing Zen meditation for decades. Practice the chant *om ah hum* (pronounced "ohm ah hoom"). For Alan, the sound and the vibration of the words as he says them makes the moment stand still in time and grounds him.

Sitting without moving can be difficult at first, so take small steps if you need to—start out with a 5-minute meditation and see how it goes. If it's tough at first, don't be too hard on yourself. The length of your meditation matters less than how well you can empty your mind. If you find a seated, quiet meditation easy, try 10, 20 or more minutes.

If this seated practice is too much to start with or simply doesn't resonate with you, don't give up on meditation and the blessings it can bring to your life! Get up and put one foot in front of the other in a walking meditation. Walk slowly, understanding that your goal isn't to "arrive" anywhere: You're just trying to be present in the moment. Leave behind any worries or cares that might be occupying your mind—before taking your first step, imagine them pouring out of your feet into the earth. During this walking meditation, the future and past aren't your concern; the focus is on the present. This isn't about power walking; it's about peacefully enjoying and focusing on each step you take with a clear and empty mind. I find that choosing a beautiful place to walk makes that path easier to follow.

MEDITATION TIPS

- Concentrate on your breathing—focus on the different sounds of the inhale and the exhale and on the different sensations of your lungs, ribs and diaphragm expanding and contracting.

- Focus on a color. (Green is one of my favorites.) "See" the color in your mind's eye and imagine it permeating every cell in your body as you "breathe the green" in and out.

- Burn incense and concentrate on the scent.

- Meditate in a group. The feeling of being in community, breathing together, can bring a different level of intention and serenity to your practice.

- Create a tranquil space to meditate in. The "Create a Tranquil Space" exercise below will help you create a retreat "outside" of your day-to-day world.

Create a Tranquil Space

Setting up a tranquil space in our homes gives us a place to go to be still, meditate, and be reminded of the blessings in our lives and what's important to us. Think of the space you create as a kind of altar. It can be any size or anywhere you like—on a mantle or little table, in the garden or on the deck. When you're deciding what you'll place on it, think about what inspires you or takes you to a deeper place within yourself. These aren't necessarily things you'd pray to—although you can choose religious icons if you wish. They can be any things that give you a lift or a sense of peace or increase the calmness and gratitude you feel in your heart. They may be things that remind you who you are and who you're choosing to be. Add elements of nature, such as a piece of driftwood from the beach or a stone you find on a hike. Take time each day to sit near your tranquil space and reflect on what you're grateful for. During the cleanse, place flowers in the space to honor the commitment you're making to your health and well-being.

THE THREE-DAY
FACE-LIFT CLEANSE

We all want to look and feel beautiful, and I believe that beauty begins and radiates from within. So the first step in transforming what's on the outside is purifying what's on the inside. It's all about rehydrating, rejuvenating your spirit, catching up on sleep and clearing out toxins that affect your skin.

The fact is, our skin is the largest organ in our bodies but is the last one to receive the nutrients and water we take in—all the other organs in the body get fed first. If we're not drinking sufficient amounts of water and eating foods packed with vitamins and minerals, we may actually be starving our skin.

When I first studied acupressure and began learning how to visually diagnose deficiencies in the body, I was amazed to see how what we put into our bodies shows up on our faces. Premature aging and lackluster or problem skin often can be traced back to the usual suspects: caffeine, alcohol, bad fats, refined flours and sugars, and so on.

The good news is that I've experienced how eating a diet of skin-nurturing nutrients, such as greens and other enzyme-rich foods, and consuming clean water and good oils and salts can enrich skin elasticity and diminish lines by flushing out the toxins that affect our appearance. And I wasn't the first to read that writing on the great wall. For 5,000 years, practitioners of traditional Chinese medicine have looked to the face as a window into the vitality of organs in the body. While studying acupressure, I learned that lines, discolorations, breakouts, and differences in skin tone or texture are indicators of internal deficiencies. Chinese face diagnosis is a complex healing art, so I won't go into a deep discussion here, but I do want to give you a small taste of how what we put into our bodies appears on our faces.

Different parts of the face are related to different internal organs. Here are some examples of what our faces might be trying to tell us:

* Dark circles or puffiness under the eyes could be an indication of overworked kidneys or adrenals, resulting from lack of sleep, dehydration, or too much partying or stress in your life.

* A lined forehead could be a warning sign of congested bowels or a gallbladder stressed by too much dairy or oily food.

* Crow's-feet might indicate that the adrenals are taxed from overuse of stimulants or living life at a nonstop pace.

* Lines over the upper lip or a larger upper lip might be pointing to an imbalance in the stomach or small intestines due to improper elimination of waste and toxins.

* Exaggerated laugh lines could be warning of a respiratory deficiency from smoking.

* Lines or blotches on the cheekbones might be indicators of an imbalance in the heart from a high-fat diet—or maybe even a broken heart.

What was true 5,000 years ago is still true today: To restore inner health and a luster to our skin, we must bring our bodies back into balance and ease stressed organs. We need to drink enough clean water, make sure we're properly eliminating waste from our bodies, and eat the right foods.

That's why I designed the Three-Day Face-Lift to be a veritable feast for the face. I combine food that's great for your skin with a healthy dose of pampering for the body and mind. (You're worth it, right?) You'll create facial spritzers, exfoliants, masks, and tea bags for the bath that protect and rejuvenate your skin and make you look and feel like you've just left the spa.

Eating healthy foods and staying hydrated may be the world's best-kept beauty secrets. So . . . you want a lift?

INCLUDE YOUR PEOPLE!

Figure out whether you want to fly solo or invite a few friends over for a face-lift party. Personally, I think you'll get an extra boost from some camaraderie and support.

If you do it as a group, get your people together one Friday and spend the evening in the kitchen mixing up the concoctions. Divvy up the responsibilities for creating the spritzer, oil, and mask, prepping the vegetables and fruit, or making the soups.

Whether you go it alone or invite friends to join you, make a commitment to shedding any negative images you have of yourself for the duration of the cleanse and devote time each day to celebrating what you find beautiful in yourself. You might just find that the positive self-reinforcement is positively addictive!

Above all, find ways to make it fun! Set up a tea-and-water bar and stock it with herbs, leaves and waters from around the world. Serve the tea in china cups, put the waters in your favorite cocktail glasses—get creative!

When to Do the Cleanse

Do this cleanse when your complexion is gray or your eyes are dull or have dark circles under them. If your skin is breaking out, dried out or weather-beaten—or if those fine lines seem not so fine anymore—it's time. If you're feeling fatigued and it's written all over your face, do this cleanse. Or do it when you just want to look and feel healthier! This is a cleanse you can do once a quarter.

What You'll See and Feel

Get ready for clear, bright eyes; glowing skin; and increased vitality. You'll look and feel calm, beautiful and vibrant. And you'll feel a renewed appreciation of yourself as a result.

JOE'S TESTIMONIAL

I'm a 36-year-old man who suddenly realized one day that I didn't have the energy that I wanted—I felt tired. People started making comments about how I looked. I had rings under my eyes, and my skin wasn't as clear as it used to be.

I hadn't been eating too badly leading up to the cleanse, but I knew I probably wasn't eating as well as I should. For instance, I'd stay away from fast foods and fried foods and breads—and I'd avoid sugary, caffeinated drinks such as sodas and iced tea because I knew they'd make me crash and affect my mood. But oftentimes, I'd let my fast metabolism give me permission to have whatever else I wanted.

Lifestyle-wise, things move at a pretty fast pace for me and my job can get stressful. But if I feel myself getting overwhelmed, I'm pretty good about taking the time I need to unplug and go for a hike or a run. But in addition to my regular job, I'm a musician. So as you might guess, I'd had my fair share of late nights partying it up with the band and the crowds. I drank more than I probably should have, and after doing a cleanse I could see the toll it had taken on my body and my face.

I had never done a cleanse before, but after some convincing, I decided to try Adina's Three-Day Face-Lift. Like I said, my life moves at a fast pace and I felt as if time was short. A three-day cleanse seemed perfect.

The first day I was really hungry. By the second day, I was still hungry, but it was different. I felt a bit off, but it wasn't the same feeling. I was skeptical about this whole cleanse thing, but I could sense my body responding, so I stayed the course. I woke up the third day rejuvenated and excited.

To get the most out of the cleanse, I made sure to keep my body moving—I walked a lot. To keep everything moving, I ended up doing a colonic as well. It wasn't an easy experience, but I realized afterward how much it contributed to this amazing rebound I was undergoing.

I looked and felt more alive. I could see a real difference in my skin. The circles under my eyes were gone and—best of all—other people noticed.

The amount of additional energy I had surprised me at first. But after speaking with Adina and doing my own research, I could see how it was directly related to what I had been eating—or rather, not eating—during the cleanse. Once day 3 was over, all I wanted was more.

I admit that before doing this cleanse I was hesitant, but I'm now a true believer in what food can do and what good food can really do. I feel healthier and have more energy, and my mind is clear.

I'll cleanse again, that much I know, because cleansing has shown me who I can be and what my body's potential is. So I'm trying to take as good care of myself as I can now. I'm much more conscious of what I eat. I'm still in the whole music scene, but I'm much more careful about how much I drink. And I'll be staying off bread products and avoiding sugar for the rest of my life . . . well, maybe a few chocolates here and there.

CLEANSE AT A GLANCE

On waking: Hot Lemon Water (see recipe on page 33)

Breakfast: Green Tonic and a shot of wheatgrass

Snack: Beauty Smoothie

Lunch: Lunch Whistle Salad

Snack: Green Tonic

Dinner: Soup of your choice

Throughout the day: Drink lemongrass, licorice root, ginger or red clover blossom teas

Special Equipment

* Blender
* Juicer
* Travel-size spray bottle
* Cheesecloth sheets
* Fine sieve

RECIPES

NOTE: Tocotrienols, lecithin grains, MSM, dulse, Udo's oil, wheatgrass and rose essential oils can be found at health-food stores. Misos are available at Asian markets. Dandelion greens are available at many grocery or specialty food stores.

GREEN TONIC

Makes 1 serving

This juice will give you a morning kick better than the one you get from a cappuccino. The enzymes in juiced vegetables break down over time, so drink your tonic the same day you make it to ensure that every drop is still chock-full of nutrients by the time you enjoy it.

1 large cucumber, peeled
5 stalks celery
1 apple, cored
3 kale leaves
4 dandelion green leaves
4 sprigs parsley
Optional garnish: a slice of fresh lemon or a squeeze of fresh lemon juice

Directions: Chop the first 6 ingredients into pieces small enough to fit through the feed tube of your juicer. Put the cucumber, celery, and apple pieces into a small bowl and the kale, dandelion green leaves, and parsley into another bowl. Run all of the ingredients through the feed tube of the juicer, alternating back and forth between the greens and the chopped vegetables and apple. If you start and end with the apple–vegetable mixture, you'll be sure to suck every juicy drop out of the greens. Serve in a large glass with a slice of lemon.

If you're new to green juices, the flavor may take some time to grow on you. If that's the case, dilute the juice with some water and squeeze in a bit more lemon juice, to taste.

BEAUTY SMOOTHIE

Makes 1 serving

This smoothie not only tastes delicious—it also makes you look delicious! MSM, or methylsulfonylmethane, is a sulfate that has been shown to improve flexibity, reduce inflammation and increase elasticity of the skin. Tocotrienols, part of the vitamin E family, have antioxidant properties that reduce free radicals in the bloodstream, which may aid in blocking skin and breast cancer. Unlike vegetables juices, which must be consumed the day they're made, this smoothie can be made the evening before you drink it to save time the following morning. Note: If you're allergic to bee stings, omit the raw honey and bee pollen.

2 cups Brazil nut or almond milk (see page 93 for recipe or buy
   almond milk at a health-food store)
1 teaspoon tocotrienols
1 teaspoon Udo's or flax oil
1 teaspoon lecithin granules
1 teaspoon green powder
1 pinch of Himalayan or Celtic sea salt
1/8 teaspoon MSM (or 1 capsule, opened up)
1 cup of your favorite berry (fresh is preferable, but frozen can work if
   the season isn't right; I recommend açaí berries)
Pinch of stevia or 2 teaspoons raw honey
1/2 teaspoon bee pollen

Directions: Add all the ingredients to your blender and mix until smooth.

ENZYME-RICH GREEN SOUP

Makes 1 serving

This is one of my favorite soups to make in any season. You can wash and prep the vegetables as early as the evening before, but blend them close to the time you'll be eating to preserve their full enzymatic power.

½ cup cucumber, peeled
1 celery stalk
1 cup arugula or spinach
½ avocado
1 cup purified water
½ clove garlic, minced
2 pinches Himalayan or Celtic sea salt
Garnish: 1 tablespoon lemon juice, minced onion, oregano and basil

Directions: Chop the first 4 ingredients into pieces small enough to be easily mixed in your blender. Place the first 7 ingredients in the blender and pulse until chopped but still chunky. Don't over-blend. Garnish with lemon juice, onion and herbs.

MELLOW BARLEY MISO SOUP

Makes 1 serving

Miso is one of my favorite wonder foods. It's high in protein, rich in vitamin B_{12}, and chock-full of 4 digestive agents that help you break down food and assimilate the nutrients. And it's got a great nutty flavor to boot!

2 cups purified water
1 tablespoon barley miso

1 tablespoon chickpea miso or red miso
½ teaspoon garlic, minced
½ teaspoon gingerroot, peeled and coarsely chopped
2 tablespoons cucumber, peeled and chopped
2 tablespoons avocado chunks
1 pinch of Himalayan or Celtic sea salt
1 pinch of powdered mustard
1 pinch of chili powder
Optional garnish: chopped avocado

Directions: Place all the ingredients into a blender. Mix until blended but not completely smooth. Heat in a medium pot on the stove until barely warm. Pour into a bowl and serve with the optional avocado garnish, if desired.

MY FAVORITE STEAMED VEGETABLES

Makes 1 serving

If you grew up thinking that steamed vegetables were boring, your family never served them this way. The dressing is almost addictive! Give yourself a break in your week and go to the farmers' market to hand-select the vegetables yourself.

Steamed Vegetables
Use any 2-cup combination of the following vegetables:
Tomatoes, quartered
Cabbage, thinly sliced
Asparagus, cut into 2-inch pieces
Sugar snap peas
Onions, cut into medium dice
Kale, chard, beet greens or any other leafy greens, torn into bite-sized pieces
Mung bean sprouts

Broccoli or cauliflower, cut into small florets
Yam, peeled and cut into medium dice

Directions: Trim off any unwanted parts of the vegetables. Add water to the pot, keeping the level below the steamer insert. Bring water to a full boil, then add the vegetables in the steamer insert. Cover pot and steam until tender. Cooking times will vary according to the vegetables you choose. When the vegetables are done, remove them from the steamer and transfer them to a large bowl. Pour dressing over the vegetables and toss well to coat.

TANGY DRESSING

2 tablespoons flax or olive oil
1 teaspoon apple cider vinegar or fresh lemon juice
Pinch of Himalayan or Celtic sea salt

Directions: Whisk ingredients together in a bowl.

THE MIGHTY ARTICHOKE

For a variation on My Favorite Steamed Vegetables, you can substitute 2 medium artichokes for the 2 cups of veggies. Artichokes are high in fiber, potassium, calcium, iron, phosphorus and other trace elements important for a balanced system, and they help clear the liver, kidneys and gallbladder as well. Here's how I cook an artichoke:

- With a pair of kitchen scissors, trim the sharp barbs off the end of the artichoke leaves.

- Cut down the stem end, and then give the artichoke a "flat top" by cutting off the top ¾ inch so the artichoke can sit in a pan with its bottom up.

- Fill a medium pot with 1 inch water. Add a pinch of Himalayan or Celtic sea salt, the juice of ½ lemon and a dash of olive oil.

- Put artichokes in the pot, bottoms up.

- Cover and bring to a boil. Reduce heat and let simmer for 45 minutes, adding water as needed.

- Remove from pot when done and allow to cool until you're able to strip off the leaves and dive in!

LUNCH WHISTLE SALAD

Makes 1 serving

The different textures of the vegetables and nuts and the contrast between the creamy avocado and tangy tomatoes and lemon dressing make this a vibrant and satisfying salad. It's quick and easy to put together too, so you can spend the bulk of your lunch break enjoying your meal, not making it.

Salad
2 cups mixed baby lettuces or the lettuce of your choice, torn into
   bite-sized pieces
1 cup sunflower sprouts
1 small cucumber, peeled and thinly sliced
½ avocado, peeled, pitted and chopped
1 apple, cored, peeled and chopped
7 soaked almonds, chopped, or 2 tablespoons pine nuts

Directions: Wash and dry the lettuce leaves. Combine the lettuce, sprouts, cucumber, avocado and apple in a salad bowl. Drizzle the dressing over the salad and toss. Serve sprinkled with almonds or pine nuts.

DRESSING

1½ tablespoons Udo's oil
1 tablespoon lemon juice
Pinch of Himalayan or Celtic sea salt
Optional: ¾ teaspoon of your favorite fresh herbs, such as parsley,
cilantro, mint, tarragon, basil, or thyme, chopped, or minced
gingerroot or cayenne pepper to taste

Directions: Whisk ingredients together in a bowl.

VEGETABLE STEW

Makes 4 servings

This filling soup really sticks to your ribs and warms you up on a cool day. You can enjoy the soup chunky or puree it in a blender (after it's cooled) if you like a smoother soup.

1 teaspoon cold-pressed extra virgin olive oil
1 cup onion, cut into small dice
5 cloves garlic, minced
1 cup fennel, cut into small dice
1 cup celery, cut into small dice
2 cups butternut squash, peeled, seeded and cut into small dice
1 cup yellow beets, cut into small dice
1 cup zucchini, cut into small dice
1 small jar of artichoke hearts, drained and cut into small pieces
7 cups purified water
⅛ teaspoon Himalayan or Celtic sea salt
Pinch of black pepper
Optional garnish: chopped cilantro, fresh lemon juice or apple cider
vinegar, pinch of hot chili paste

Directions: Heat oil in large saucepan over medium heat. Add onions. Sauté for about 5 minutes, until golden, and then add garlic,
fennel, celery, butternut squash, yellow beets, zucchini and artichoke hearts and sauté for another 5 minutes. Add purified water,
salt and pepper and bring to a boil. Reduce heat and simmer for
about 30 minutes until veggies are tender. Ladle into a bowl, season with optional garnish if desired, and enjoy.

Cleanse-Boosting Activities

Pamper Your Face
Boost the rejuvenating effects of face-friendly foods by scheduling
a facial or a Shiatsu face massage, spritzing your face with
rose-infused oil throughout the day and doing an exfoliating or
rehydrating mask. After trying these easy, nourishing recipes with
natural ingredients, you may decide to leave commercial creams
behind.

FACIAL SPRITZ

Makes 4 ounces

I love this rehydrating spritz—the combination of water and essential oils is totally reviving. The travel-size bottle fits easily into any
tote or handbag, so I can bring them with me wherever I go.

½ cup purified water
2 drops rose essential oil

Directions: Put water into travel-size spritzer bottle and add rose
essential oil. Put the cap back on and start spritzing!

FACIAL SCRUB

Makes 1 application

The exfoliating properties of the gritty cornmeal leave your face invigorated and glowing.

2 tablespoons whole-fat organic plain yogurt
2 tablespoons ground cornmeal

Directions: Mix the yogurt and cornmeal into a paste. Gently rub the mixture into your skin in small circles, starting at the chin and working up to the cheeks and forehead, and then the hairline. Rinse with warm water and dab skin dry.

FINGER-LICKING-GOOD MASK

Makes 1 application

The fats in the avocado are amazing natural moisturizers for your skin. This mask is especially cool and soothing after a day in the wind or sun or when dry winter weather has left your face feeling parched.

1 avocado, peeled and pitted

Directions: After you peel and pit the avocado, take a bite . . . lick your fingers—go ahead and give it to yourself! Then mash the rest of the avocado into a soft paste. Massage into your face, using circular motions. Leave on for 2 minutes, and then wash off with warm water.

Baby Your Body

Steep your entire body in an herbal tea soak (see recipe below). The essential oils of the herbs in the tea bags have a relaxing effect.

When you're brewing in the tub, breathe through your nose and imagine exhaling any stress or negative feelings carried over from the day and inhaling feelings of harmony and peace. Don't have a bathtub? No problem. Pour boiling water into a pot, add the herbs, lean over the pot, steam your face with a towel draped over your head and the pot, and breathe deeply.

To give the rest of your body a lovely glow, massage in coconut oil from your shoulders to your toes to seal in moisture after bathing or showering.

TEA BAG FOR THE BATH

Makes 3 tea bags, enough for 3 baths

The lavender and chamomile here make for a calming, soothing way to end your day. You can find the dried flowers and leaves at many health-food markets. I pop a tea bag into a hot bath, light a few candles and feel the stress of the day melt away.

¼ cup dried chamomile flowers
¼ cup dried lavender flowers
2 sheets of cheesecloth, cut into 6 equal pieces
3 pieces of cotton string or twine

Directions: Mix the dried flowers together in a small bowl. Layer 2 of the cut cheesecloth squares on top of each other. Put ⅓ of the flower mixture into the center of the cheesecloth square. Lift the 4 ends of the cloth together and twist, sealing the flower buds in the center of the bundle. The buds will expand when submerged in the bath, so leave room for that expansion. Tie up the bundle with a piece of string. Repeat the process for the next 2 bags.

Pinpoint the Fountain of Youth

Feel as if you've had a little nip and tuck without going under the knife . . . with Shiatsu facial massage. Done over time, in combination with a healing diet, it can erase years off your face. During the therapy, pressure is placed on different energy meridians on your face and body. The pressure clears energy blockages and helps release toxins that lead to premature aging from the body.

"SOME LIKE IT RAW" CLEANSE (5 TO 7 DAYS)

f you've never "gone raw" before, it might sound daunting. You might think, *Raw food for five to seven days? Please! I want flavor . . . I want a satisfying meal.* But one taste of the recipes in this chapter is going to wipe out any reservations you might have about a vegan, raw-foods diet. You'll be surprised at how satisfying and flavorful the food is—and it's incredibly healing and nourishing for your body as well.

Raw vegan foods have little or no saturated fats and no trans fats, and they're packed with essential nutrients such as potassium, magnesium, folates, and vitamins A, C and E. They contain a lot of water and fiber, which helps flush the intestines of waste and toxins that make us feel lethargic. They also have the perfect amount of natural enzymes to efficiently break down their own sugars, proteins, fats, carbohydrates and fibers into digestible particles and increase our metabolism.

That's important, because we're each born with finite reserves of the enzymes that fuel every chemical reaction in our body, including cell division, immunity, energy production and brain activity. When we cook food at temperatures higher than 118 degrees Fahrenheit, we lose 30% to 50% of its vitamins and destroy its natural enzymes. Without those natural enzymes, we have to tap into the digestive enzymes our body produces, which depletes our reserves and requires more energy—energy that could be better spent building and healing the body. When we eat raw foods, we conserve our digestive enzymes, which ultimately helps slow the aging process and fend off disease.

Sprouted seeds and nuts are a major feature in raw-food recipes. When we soak seeds and nuts and force them to sprout, they enter a huge growth spurt to begin turning into a plant—that's why they're referred to as live foods. They're packed with a level of proteins, amino acids and chlorophyll that you just don't find in cooked foods—all of which help regenerate cells and boost immunity. Fermented foods, which aid in digestion, are also part of a raw-food diet, so you'll see them included in several of the recipes as well.

When I look back, there were a couple of things that got me hooked on the raw movement. First was how incredibly vibrant raw foodists looked—these people were radiant. Second was the food Chef Juliano served as his San Francisco restaurant Raw. The flavors and textures were amazing; the food woke up my entire palate and totally sated my appetite.

I wanted to download what was happening in his kitchen, so I landed a job there and began exploring the power of living foods. Preparing food this way was like learning a new language—it opened my eyes to new culinary possibilities. While I worked there, I ate 100% raw and met many other raw-foodists. We were each struck by the amount of energy we had and how our skin glowed. The thing that surprised me most was that my eyes became a lighter shade of blue.

Ponce de León got it wrong when he traveled the world searching for the fountain of youth—it's been hidden in our kitchens all along.

"UNCOOKING"

Because raw food isn't heated above 118 degrees Fahrenheit, a raw-foods chef taps into a different set of cooking techniques:

- Blending soups, sauces and beverages
- Juicing fruits and vegetables
- Sprouting legumes, seeds and grains
- Fermenting vegetables, nuts, beans, grains and seeds
- Soaking nuts or dried fruits
- Dehydrating foods

When to Do the Cleanse

If you're run down and in need of a total vitality recharge, it's time to do this cleanse. If you're bloated and nothing you eat seems to be moving through you; if you feel stuck physically, emotionally, or mentally or need a spiritual lift; if you want a serious boost in how youthful and healthy you feel; if your skin is looking gray and you want to get a glow, do this cleanse.

NOTE: Because some people find it hard to give up the comfort of warm foods during the winter, I recommend doing this cleanse in warmer-weather months.

What You'll See and Feel

As you free your body of stored fat, wastes and toxins, it has an easier time recalibrating to its ideal weight. Not only will you shed pounds but also your skin will look younger and healthier and your eyes will be brighter. You'll feel clearer-headed and have a greater sense of peace and balance. And with the boost in energy you'll get from eating raw foods, you'll be able to break off any long-term engagement you might have had with the snooze button on your alarm clock.

JUSTIN'S TESTIMONIAL

Two years ago, I began eating a raw, vegan diet as a last-ditch effort to get relief from some chronic health problems. For the 2 previous years, I'd had severe psoriasis, with red, itchy blisters covering my arms, calves and torso. In addition, the muscles of my lower body, hands and lower back were in constant spasm and pain. My physician had prescribed a host of conventional, drug-based treatments to relieve my symptoms, but none were successful.

At the time, I was an exercise therapist at Egoscue in San Francisco, California. The founder, Pete Egoscue, referred me to Robert Young, PhD, DSc, ND, after hearing about my struggle. Dr. Young is a microbiologist and author of The pH Miracle, *who'd been doing research into something called "new biology" for more than 30 years. Pete's wife had cured herself of breast cancer by following his dietary and lifestyle recommendations, so I was hopeful he'd be able to help me too.*

I went to one of Dr. Young's 3-day retreats where he presented his findings about why an alkaline diet was critical to restoring balance in the body. As I listened, I began to look at health and disease in a completely different light. New biology looks at the symptoms of disease as the body's compensation mechanisms to regain and maintain internal balance, especially the homeostasis of our blood pH. After decades of research, he found that the key to bringing the body back into homeostasis was a combination of a diet of primarily raw, vegan, organic, alkaline foods and a balanced lifestyle. The more I heard, the more confident I became that Dr. Young had the answer I'd been looking for.

While I was there, I had a live blood analysis done. Dr. Young was actually able to tell from my lab results that I was experiencing severe muscle spasms, circulatory problems, skin problems and emotional issues. And he gave me a plan for getting my body back into balance, which included a diet of alkaline foods such as salads, sprouts, vegetables and vegetable juices.

Up to that point, I'd been on a standard high-calorie fitness diet that included lots of meat proteins, protein powders, carbs and workout stimulants such as caffeine. Ever since seventh grade, I'd been seriously working out, lifting weights for at least 2 hours a day. I'd totally avoided vegetables for 6 years because they were low calorie and I was trying to bulk up.

At the same time, I was always overstressing my body. I was dealing with a lot of emotional stress from a relationship that had ended and worked long hours and pushed my body to the limit with my workouts as a way to deal with it. The emotional and physical stress my body was under, combined with the workout stimulants, kept my body in a constant fight-or-flight response mode. The acid levels in my body were skyrocketing as result, and I knew it all had to stop.

When I switched to an alkaline diet, the effects were unbelievable— the itching from the psoriasis stopped on the first day; by the third day, the blisters had healed; and by day 7 it was completely gone. I was psoriasis-free for the first time in years. The chronic pain I'd been experiencing took 2 months to fade away, but I remember the instant I realized it was gone: I was really getting into a cricket game on television and it suddenly occurred to me I was thinking about something other than pain. It was miraculous.

The transition to a primarily raw, alkaline diet wasn't easy. I faced intense cravings for carbohydrates initially—breaking down in the late afternoon and bingeing on peanut butter, chocolate, chicken and rice, etc.—but the cravings eventually subsided as my motivation to be pain-free drove me onward.

I noticed that eating a really clean diet had a big impact on my mental and emotional states too. I had so much more clarity that when an issue came up in my life, there was no burying it—I had to confront *and deal with it. To cultivate inner peace, I began practicing Vedic meditation. That became a big part of the healing equation for me and helped me stick to an alkaline diet.*

Today, my energy and mental clarity have never been better, and I feel completely present in the moment. When I compare the level of energy I had and the massive quantities of food I'd eaten before with the energy I have and the amount of food I eat now, it blows me away. When you're eating foods that contain the nutrients your body really needs, you need so much less of it.

My experience was so dramatic that I changed careers to become a nutritional microscopy consultant so I could help others the way Dr. Young helped me. I absolutely recommend a raw, vegan, alkaline diet to anyone who's interested in dramatically improving his or her health.

CLEANSE AT A GLANCE

On waking: Hot Lemon Water (see recipe on page 33)

Breakfast: Selection from the breakfast options

Lunch: Selection from the lunch options

Snack: Tea and a shot of wheatgrass

Dinner: Selection from the dinner options

Before bed: A cup of chamomile, valerian root, or any other calming, sleepy-time tea

---

Special Equipment

* High-speed blender
* Juicer
* Food processor
* Spiralizer

✳ Fine sieve or nut-milk bag
✳ Dehydrator*

RECIPES

NOTE: Cacao nibs, flax oil, agave, stevia, green powder and wheatgrass are available at health-food stores. Young coconuts, chickpea miso, nori sheets, umeboshi vinegar, kimchee and daikon radishes are available at Asian markets.

Breakfast Choices

HEAVENLY GREEN JUICE

Makes one 16-ounce serving

I always start my raw cleanse off with a green juice packed with all the green power I can get my hands on—it's a great way to get myself back on track. The chlorophyll in each sip is calming, immunity-boosting, and cleansing for your blood. Remember, it's best to use a juicer, but if you don't have one and aren't sure if you're ready to buy one, you can use a blender for the juice recipes (see instructions on page 15).

1/2 head celery (about 4 large celery sticks)
6 leaves rainbow chard or beet greens
1/2 apple, cored

*The majority of the recipes for this cleanse don't require a dehydrator. But because so many of my clients have made raw foods a regular part of their ongoing diet after doing this cleanse, I have included a few recipes here that call for a dehydrator or have dehydration as a cooking option, in case you're feeling adventurous and want to totally jump onto the raw-foods bandwagon.

2 cups pea sprouts
1 small cucumber
2 tablespoons fresh lemon juice

Directions: Chop the first 5 ingredients into pieces small enough to fit into the feeder tube of your juicer. Juice the fruit and vegetables, starting with the celery and ending with the cucumber to ensure that you get as much juice as possible out of the sprouts. Stir in lemon juice. Add water as needed to make a 16-ounce serving.

LIVER-CLEANSE SMOOTHIE*

Makes 4 servings

I adapted this recipe from work I did with Dr. David Jubb of Jubb's Longevity on the Lower East Side of New York City. The lemon and oil detoxify the liver while boosting the immune system. It's a surprisingly delicious way to start your day.

2 large lemons or 1 grapefruit, peel and white pith removed, cut into large pieces
1 small apple or pear, cored, peeled and chopped into large dice
3 tablespoons flax oil
¼ teaspoon of Himalayan or Celtic sea salt
Optional: pinch of cayenne
2 cups purified water

Directions: Put all ingredients into a blender and process until smooth. Pour into a glass and add water to make 16 ounces as needed.

---

*Denotes recipes that are appropriate for breaking the stringent cleanses—the Urban Revitalizer, Winter Wake-Up and Green Buzz.

ALMOND MILK†

Makes 2 servings

This easy-to-make milk is great in your tea and it's an important ingredient in several recipes in this book. Almonds are rich in calcium, iron and phosphorus. I recommend buying raw almonds from the farmers' market, because almonds at grocery stores have been pasteurized, killing some of their nutrients. For variety, you can experiment by substituting hazelnuts, pumpkinseeds or Brazil nuts for the almonds. You can adjust the flavorings to your palate. Add cinnamon and vanilla and a few dates for a real treat.

1 cup raw almonds, soaked overnight
4 cups coconut water or purified water
Pinch of Himalayan or Celtic sea salt
Optional: pinch of cinnamon or vanilla bean seeds

Directions: Process all ingredients in a blender until smooth; strain through fine sieve or nut-milk bag. Rinse blender; pour milk back into blender with the pinch of salt and your choice of the cinnamon or vanilla (if you choose to use them); and blend until all are incorporated. Pour half of the milk into a glass and enjoy. The remaining milk will keep for 2 days in the refrigerator.

GREEN APPLE PORRIDGE*

Makes 2 servings

This porridge is packed with pectin, fiber and omega-3 fatty acids; and the flax seeds in the recipe make this porridge an effective intestinal broom. Soaking the almonds overnight starts the sprouting process, boosts the enzyme count and makes them easier to digest.

Try using extra-green sour apples for an extra dose of vitamin C and malic acid, which helps cleanse the gallbladder.

2 green apples, cored, peeled and chopped into large dice
1/4 cup almonds, soaked overnight
2 black mission figs
1 tablespoon flaxseeds
1/4 teaspoon fresh ginger, peeled and finely minced
Pinch of Himalayan or Celtic sea salt

Directions: Process all the ingredients in a food processor with the S blade until smooth. Spoon into a bowl and enjoy.

MY FAVORITE SWEET YOGURT†

Makes 2 servings

Walnuts don't just resemble a brain—they're great brain food too. So if you need to start your day on your toes mentally, give this recipe a try. This yogurt is so creamy and delicious, you'll think it's made with dairy, and the fruit adds the perfect touch of sweetness.

1 cup walnuts, soaked overnight
1/2 cup water
2 teaspoons fresh lemon or grapefruit juice
2 figs, soaked overnight
1/2 teaspoon agave syrup or pinch of stevia
1/4 cup of your choice of fresh berries, apple or pear (core and peel apple or pear if you choose either of them)

Directions: Process all ingredients in blender until creamy. Transfer 1 serving to a bowl and enjoy. Second serving will keep in the refrigerator for 2 days.

BUDDHABERRY SMOOTHIE

Makes 2 servings

I love this smoothie for breakfast or a late-afternoon snack. You can add any super green powder to this recipe. There are great green powders out there, such as Pure Synergy and Greener Grasses, that boost the chlorophyll content even further by including a mix of wheatgrass, barley grass, alfalfa, chlorella, and numerous other greens. Green powders are available at health-food stores.

2 cups coconut water
2 teaspoons almond butter
½ cup berries of your choice (I love blueberries!)
1 or 2 scoops of protein powder (choose a non-whey, non-soy-based powder)

Directions: Put all ingredients into a blender and process until smooth. Pour 1 serving into a glass and enjoy. The remaining serving will keep in the refrigerator for 1 day.

Lunch Choices

RED PEPPER COLLARD WRAP†

Makes 4 servings

Collard wraps are your new best friends when you pack them full of delicious pâté. This is a satisfying lunch and easy to pack up when you're on the go.

1 cup fresh cilantro, chopped
1 cup arugula, chopped

1 cup raw macadamia nuts
1 large cucumber, peeled and chopped into medium dice
1 cup sugar snap peas
½ clove garlic, minced
2 tablespoons fresh lemon juice
⅛ teaspoon Himalayan or Celtic sea salt, or more to taste
Pinch of cayenne
2 medium red or yellow bell peppers, tops removed and seeded
4 large collard green leaves
Optional: 2 tablespoons olives, chopped

Directions: Process first 10 ingredients in a food processor with the S blade until it's incorporated into a coarse paste. Roll up ¼ of the filling into each collard green leaf with a sprinkle of the optional olives.

MEZUNTE BURRITO †

Makes 4 servings

Cabbage leaves serve as the tortillas in this raw take on a burrito—it's high in calcium and does a great job cleansing the digestive tract. The filling has a little kick that goes perfectly with a dollop of guacamole or the raw pepper jack cheese. If you're not a cabbage fan, substitute green or red leaf lettuce.

½ cup walnuts, soaked overnight
½ cup pumpkinseeds, soaked overnight
2 tablespoons fresh lime juice
¼ teaspoon umeboshi vinegar
½ teaspoon cumin
1 tablespoon onion, chopped
½ cup cilantro, chopped
½ teaspoon jalapeño, seeded and chopped

4 cabbage leaves
1 avocado, peeled, pitted and chopped
1 small tomato, chopped
1 tablespoon green olives, pitted and chopped
1 cup romaine, shredded
Lime wedges

Directions: Process the first 6 ingredients in a food processor until nuts and seeds resemble a coarse meal. Transfer to a large bowl and stir in cilantro and jalapeño. Scoop 2 heaping tablespoons of pâté into a cabbage leaf. Top with chopped avocado, tomato, olives, shredded romaine and a squeeze of lime. Roll up cabbage leaf, burrito-style, and enjoy.

TASMANIAN TABOULI[†]

Makes 2 servings

This is a delicious salad from my childhood. Broccoli is a great source of calcium, and the hemp seeds—the substitute for bulgur wheat in this raw tabouli—naturally flush the intestine. Top with tahini sauce and a few dried currants if you'd like to add a little something extra to the dish.

2 large broccoli heads, well washed and chopped into large dice
⅛ teaspoon Himalayan or Celtic sea salt
3 tablespoons hemp seeds
Juice of 4 lemons
¼ cup olive oil
2 teaspoons fresh mint, minced
Generous pinch of fresh ground black pepper
2 cups tomatoes, seeded and diced
1 cucumber, peeled, seeded and chopped into small dice

3 tablespoons olives of your choice, pitted and chopped
Optional: 2 tablespoons dried currants

Put broccoli pieces into a food processor and chop until pieces are the size of rice grains. Transfer the broccoli to a large bowl and add salt, massaging it into the broccoli to help the fibers break down. Add hemp seeds. In a separate bowl, whisk together the lemon juice, olive oil, mint, salt and pepper until smooth. Pour the dressing over the broccoli mixture, toss and let marinate for 1 hour. Add tomatoes, cucumber, olives and optional currants. Toss and serve.

FALAFEL WITH LEMON TAHINI SAUCE[†]

Makes 4 servings

Falafel balls are easy to make and great to take on the go, so make a batch and keep them in the fridge. They're dehydrated, so they're much lower in fat than their deep-fried cousins. You can eat them in a lettuce leaf or dip them into tahini sauce on their own.

Falafel
1 cup pecans, soaked overnight, or sprouted mung beans (see page
   149 for sprouting instructions)
1 cup walnuts, soaked overnight
1/2 cup jicama or cucumber, peeled and chopped into medium dice
1/2 cup sesame seeds, ground
1 cup parsley, minced
1/2 cup cilantro, minced
1 teaspoon garlic, minced
1 teaspoon cumin
Pinch of black pepper
1/2 teaspoon Himalayan or Celtic sea salt
2 tablespoons olive oil

Blend pecans or sprouted mung beans, walnuts, and jicama or cucumber to a fine meal in a food processor. Transfer to a bowl and mix in the remaining ingredients by hand. Roll spoonfuls of the mixture into 1-inch balls and flatten each ball with your thumb. Place flattened disks into a dehydrator at 118 degrees Fahrenheit for 6 to 8 hours.

LEMON TAHINI SAUCE

3 tablespoons purified water
1/2 cup raw tahini
1/3 cup fresh lemon juice
1/3 cup red bell pepper, chopped
1/4 teaspoon Himalayan or Celtic sea salt
1/4 teaspoon agave syrup
1 tablespoon olive oil
Optional: 1 teaspoon garlic, minced

Directions. In a blender, process all ingredients until smooth and creamy.

CHOPPED SALAD WITH GODDESS DRESSING†

Makes 4 servings

If you're dragging by midday, this spicy salad dressing is sure to open your eyes! Add a dollop of "cheese" (from page 109) if you'd like a more filling, protein-rich salad. The raw sauerkraut can be purchased at health food stores.

Chopped Salad

1 head romaine lettuce, torn into bite-sized pieces
1/2 cup cucumber, thinly sliced

1 cup cherry tomatoes, halved

1½ cups sprouts of your choice (use at least ½ cup bean, pea or lentil sprouts)

1 cup leafy greens such as arugula, spinach or mâche

½ avocado, pitted, peeled and chopped into small dice

4 tablespoons raw sauerkraut

Directions: Place all ingredients in a large bowl and toss. Place ¼ of the salad on a plate, drizzle with the goddess dressing, and enjoy.

DRESSING

1 cup macadamia nuts

⅓ cup purified water

1 tablespoon lemon juice

1 tablespoon apple cider

Pinch of black pepper

Directions: Process nuts into fine meal in a food processor. Add the rest of the ingredients and process until smooth. Use to dress the salad and store the remaining dressing in the refrigerator.

FISH-FRIENDLY SUSHI†

Makes 6 servings

I can't go very long without sushi, so I love this recipe. It hits the spot and makes me feel as if I'm eating the real thing. You can substitute any nut for the sunflower seeds, but the seeds make this lower in fat. If you want to make the sushi in advance, place dry, washed lettuce leaves on the nori sheets before filling them—they'll serve as a barrier and keep the nori fresh and firm while you wait to eat.

RICE

---

2 cups sunflower seeds or almonds, soaked overnight
1 cup sunflower sprouts or sprouted mung bean (see page 149 for
*   sprouting instructions)*
⅓ cup lemon juice
⅓ cup cilantro
½ cup carrot, cut into small dice
1 teaspoon minced gingerroot
Pinch of salt
½ teaspoon ume plum vinegar

Directions: Process all ingredients in blender into a grain-sized meal.

FILLINGS OF YOUR CHOICE

The sky's the limit when you think about what you'd like to use as a filling in your sushi. Some of my favorites follow. Grating the vegetables or julienning them will make it easier to slice the sushi into pieces when you're done.

Daikon radish
Avocado
Cucumber
Sweet red or yellow bell peppers
Sprouts
Sesame seeds
Fresh herbs
Kimchee

WRAPPER

6 nori sheets

Directions: Spread "rice" to desired thickness in rectangle covering the bottom ⅓ of the long side of a nori sheet. Lay the fillings of choice in lengthwise strips atop the "rice." Be careful not to add too many fillings or you may struggle to roll the nori sheet. Begin tightly rolling the nori, starting from the filled end. When you come to the end of the nori sheet, wet your finger, run it along the loose end of the sheet and then press this end into the roll to seal it. To slice the nori roll, use a sharp knife and cut slowly, exerting only enough pressure to cut while being careful not to squash the roll. Keep your knife clean for easier cutting!

Dinner Choices

ANGEL HAIR PESTO

Makes 6 servings

You'll be surprised to see how similar spiralized squash is to actual pasta. Thick, straight squash works best. If you'd like, you can also use butternut squash or daikon radish. The pesto recipe yields more than needed for the "pasta," so you can use the remaining pesto on steamed or blanched vegetables or store it in a closed container in the refrigerator for two days.

"Pasta"
2 yellow summer squash, whole, with ends removed
2 zucchini squash, whole, with ends removed
1 cup tomato, chopped into medium dice (green and red heirlooms are best)

1 tablespoon pine nuts
¼ cup fresh lemon juice
½ cup parsley, minced
½ cup basil, minced
Optional garnish: additional squeeze of fresh lemon juice; 8 Moroccan
    olives, pitted and chopped

Directions: Shred the squash using a vegetable spiralizer. Toss the squash with the remaining ingredients in a large bowl. Add pesto, several tablespoons at a time, tossing in between, until you get the desired taste. Add optional squeeze of lemon juice and the olives, toss, and serve.

PESTO

1 cup pine nuts
1 cup basil leaves, destemmed
1 cup parsley leaves, destemmed
1 clove garlic, minced
4 tablespoons olive oil
Pinch of Himalayan or Celtic sea salt

Directions: Place all ingredients in a food processor using an S blade, and blend until you get a smooth consistency. Store unused pesto in an airtight container in the refrigerator.

MICHELLA'S RAWVIOLIS†

Makes 2 servings

This is a delicious and creative way to make raw raviolis. The cashews are an excellent source of protein and add a lovely cheesy flavor that contrasts with the kick of the olives. If you'd like to experiment with a dehydrator in this recipe, you can cook the filled raw-violis in a dehydrator at 118 degrees Fahrenheit for 2½ to 3 hours—before adding the tomato sauce—to warm them.

Filling

1 cup cashews
½ cup jicama or cucumber, peeled and chopped into large dice
2 tablespoons fresh lemon juice
1 teaspoon chopped basil
⅛ teaspoon Himalayan or Celtic sea salt
Pinch of black pepper
Pinch of cayenne
¼ cup green olives, pitted and diced
2 tablespoons fresh basil, minced
1 teaspoon fresh parsley or oregano, minced
2 medium zucchini, cut into thin, lengthwise slices using a mandoline
   or vegetable peeler
¾ teaspoon Himalayan or Celtic sea salt

Directions: In a food processor, blend first 7 ingredients into a smooth paste. Transfer to a bowl and mix in the olives, basil, and parsley or oregano. Cut zucchini into very thin slices using a mandoline or a large vegetable peeler; lay them in a single layer atop paper towels. Sprinkle the zucchini with the salt and let sit for 20 minutes—this will soften the zucchini and make it easier to roll. Brush salt off zucchini. Place a tablespoon of pâté atop the end of each zucchini slice and roll.

TOMATO SAUCE

Raw tomato sauces are quite simple. Remember that it is always about quality ingredients. Start with really ripe and delicious organic tomatoes, a little bit of red pepper, a bit of olive oil and some herbs. You may wonder why you ever cooked a sauce before. Note: if you'd like a thicker sauce, seed the tomatoes before dicing.

4 large ripe tomatoes, chopped into large dice
1/2 cup sun-dried tomatoes, soaked for 2 to 3 hours
1/4 cup olive oil
1 sweet red pepper, chopped into large dice
1 tablespoon fresh basil, chopped
1/2 teaspoon oregano, chopped
1/8 small clove garlic, minced
1 teaspoon Himalayan or Celtic sea salt
Pinch of black pepper
Pinch of cayenne
Pinch of ground clove

Add all ingredients to the blender and process until smooth. Spoon sauce over rawviolis and serve.

TOMATO STACKS†

Makes 2 servings

Pine nuts give this dish a nice buttery taste and are high in protein and minerals. It's incredibly easy to make as a snack or meal. It gets rave reviews when I serve it as passed hors d'oeuvres at parties. If you can't find jicama, substitute thin slices of peeled cucumber, cut on a diagonal.

1 cup macadamia or pine nuts
1/4 cup fresh lemon juice
1/2 teaspoon Himalayan or Celtic sea salt
1/3 cup basil, chopped
1/3 cup cilantro, chopped

1 tablespoon marjoram, chopped

2 tablespoons olives of your choice, pitted and chopped

3 large ripe tomatoes of your choice, cut crosswise into ¼-inch-thick
   slices

½ jicama, peeled and sliced thinly on a mandoline

1 avocado, pitted, peeled and chopped into small dice

⅓ cup sprouts of your choice

Garnish: lemon wedges

Directions: Process nuts in food processor until ground into fine meal. Add lemon juice and salt, pulsing a few times to combine. Transfer mixture to a separate bowl and add herbs and olives. Spread nut filling onto a tomato slice, then place a slice of jicama over the filling. Spread more nut filling over the jicama and then top with avocado pieces and sprouts. Transfer to a plate, garnished with lemon wedges.

KALE–AVOCADO SALAD[†]

Makes 4 servings

Get your chlorophyll fix! I adapted this recipe from one I learned at the Tree of Life Rejuvenation Center. If you've never tried kale like this before, give it a whirl. The creamy avocado, cool tomato and tangy olive combination make this salad a crowd-pleaser.

1 head kale, cut into chiffonade

1 cup arugula

2 tablespoons fresh lemon or lime juice

½ teaspoon Himalayan or Celtic sea salt

2 avocados, diced

2 teaspoons Brazil nuts or sunflower seeds, ground

2 radishes, chopped

1 cup tomato, chopped
3 tablespoons olives of your choice, pitted and chopped
Optional: dash of cayenne

Toss first 5 ingredients together in large mixing bowl with your hands, squeezing as you mix to wilt the kale, break down the fibers, and coat the leaves with avocado. Add the remaining ingredients and mix together. Spoon a serving onto a plate and enjoy.

"MOVE OVER, ANDY WARHOL" CREAM OF TOMATO SOUP[†]

Makes 2 servings

If Andy had known how amazing a raw tomato soup could taste, he might never have created that painting . . .

4 large ripe tomatoes, cut into large dice
2 medium carrots, cut into small dice
½ avocado, pitted and peeled, or 5 raw macadamia nuts
1 cucumber, peeled and cut into large dice
1 cup sprouts of your choice
1 tablespoon fresh lemon juice
½ cup parsley, chopped
Pinch of ground clove
Pinch of celery seed
Pinch of Himalayan or Celtic sea salt
Fresh ground black pepper to taste

Directions: In a blender, process all ingredients until smooth and creamy. Chill for 1 to 2 hours, and then serve.

COOL CARROT SOUP

Makes 1 serving

This is a fun twist on the usual carrot soup. The power of carrots and pine nuts can't be denied, and I really like the marriage of the sweetness with the heat of the jalapeño.

1 cup carrot juice, from approximately 6 large carrots
1 cup cucumber juice, from 1 large cucumber
¼ cup pine nuts
1 small clove garlic, peeled and minced
1 teaspoon jalapeño, seeded and chopped
2 teaspoons fresh lime juice
Pinch of nutmeg

Directions: In a blender, process all ingredients until smooth and creamy. Pour serving into a bowl and enjoy.

MAGIC MINESTRONE†

Makes 4 servings

This is not your typical minestrone from the old country, but it tastes great and has lots of flavor. *Mangia, mangia, mangia!*

4 medium tomatoes, plus 1 cup tomato, diced
2 carrots, cut into large dice
1½ tablespoons miso
2 cups purified water
1 cup mixed vegetables of your choice, cut into small dice (zucchini, fennel, sugar snap peas, avocado, snow peas, etc.)
2 tablespoons fresh parsley, finely chopped

1 teaspoon olive oil
2 tablespoons basil, finely chopped
2 teaspoons dried Italian spices
1 small clove garlic, peeled and minced
Pinch of cayenne
Himalayan or Celtic sea salt to taste
Fresh ground pepper to taste

Directions: In a blender, process the 4 tomatoes, carrots, miso and water until smooth. Transfer the mixture into a bowl and add remaining ingredients. Stir to incorporate. Pour a serving into a bowl and enjoy.

Side Dish Choices

NOTE: Each of these recipes makes great a flavor addition to the lunch or dinner menus. Throw a dollop of primo pâté onto the tabouli. Add guacamole to the burrito. And the "cheese" is a great addition to the rawviolis.

RAW PEPPER JACK "CHEESE"

Makes 4 servings

Not even the cows would guess this wasn't actual cheese. It's a great spread on raw crackers, and makes a nice dip for veggies or a yummy filling for lettuce leaves.

1 cup Brazil nuts
3 tablespoons fresh lemon juice
Dash of umeboshi vinegar
2 teaspoons cilantro, chopped

5 tablespoons purified water
Pinch of cayenne
Couple of pinches of black pepper

Directions: Grind Brazil nuts into a fine meal in a food processor. Add remaining ingredients and blend until smooth. You can slowly add more water to adjust the consistency.

GREAT GUAC†

Makes 4 servings

Avocados are gifts from the gods. In addition to being delicious, they're carb-free and contain good fats, so they're often the heart and soul of raw-foods dishes. You can use this guacamole as a dip for veggies or raw crackers, or just grab a spoon and dive in!

2 avocados, pitted, peeled and mashed
Juice of 1 lime
1 clove garlic, minced
1 tablespoon red onion, chopped
1 teaspoon jalapeño or habañero chili, seeded and chopped
2 tablespoons cilantro, chopped
⅛ teaspoon Himalayan or Celtic sea salt

Directions: Mix all ingredients together in a medium bowl.

PRIMO PÂTÉ

Makes 4 servings

I like this recipe because it's easy to make, satisfying and full of flavor. I have it on hand in my refrigerator at all times.

2 cups walnuts
1 cup cucumber, peeled and cut into cubes
1/4 cup green olives, pitted and chopped
1 cup sprouts (I recommend sunflower sprouts for this recipe)
1 scallion
1 clove garlic, chopped
1/4 cup purified water
Pinch of Himalayan or Celtic sea salt
Pinch of fresh ground black pepper

Directions: In a food processor with the S blade process walnuts into a fine meal. Add remaining ingredients and blend until mixture forms a thick paste.

CHOCONUT "MILK"

Makes 1 serving

If you've just got to have something sweet to get you through the day, try this healthier version of chocolate milk. Instructions for opening a young coconut are on page 160. For a thicker, more filling drink you can include the flesh from the coconut.

Water from 1 young coconut
1 teaspoon cacao nibs
Pinch of agave nectar or stevia

Directions: Put all ingredients into a blender and process for 10 seconds. Pour into a glass and enjoy.

Cleanse-Boosting Activities

Get Out of Your Head and Into Your Body!

Look for a Qigong class in your area. *Qi* means "breath" and *gong* means "work." Qigong, or energy cultivation, is an aspect of Chinese medicine incorporating different breathing patterns with various physical postures and motions of the body. It is incredibly rejuvenating and therapeutic. The philosophy claims that humanity and nature are inseparable and that this practice can help us access higher energy and achieve a highly relaxed and tranquil mind–body state.

Explore!

After you've sampled a few of the recipes and seen how delectable raw foods can be, you may want to book a reservation at a raw-foods restaurant in your city or pop on over to the local bookstore and check out all the raw-foods cookbooks.

Surprise your friends at your next dinner party by serving an exotic raw-foods meal. Get everyone involved in preparing the meal—part of the fun of going raw is getting in there and creating meals in an entirely new way.

Feeling Raw? Let It Go

Holding in negative emotions—anger, pain, resentment, and so on—ultimately takes a toll on our body and our spirit. So if you find yourself carrying around some emotional baggage and want to lighten your load, give this lesson in forgiveness a try. Find a quiet place where you won't be interrupted and get into a comfortable position seated or lying down. Take a few deep, clearing breaths. Think about the situation that feels a bit raw and about exactly what was so upsetting—it could be something another person said or did or maybe something you said or did. If someone hurt you, visualize talking to that person about how you feel—if you're angry or upset with yourself, visualize talking yourself through that. When you've said your piece, say this affirmation aloud: "These feelings are no longer serving me. I release them to set my body and soul free. I forgive (name), I forgive (name), I forgive (name)." As you say this affirmation, imagine opening up the internal vault of all that pent-up negative energy and releasing it into the wind. Letting go can lighten your spirit, and because negative emotions end up affecting us physically—often manifesting in disease—you'll be giving yourself the gift of health as well.

THE KARMA CLEANSE
(5 TO 10 DAYS)

When we throw the word *karma* around today, we're usually referring to someone getting payback for something he or she has done, good or bad. But if we flip back through the history books, that wasn't what the rishis in India had in mind when they defined the concept of karma more than 5,000 years ago. They didn't see karmas as good or bad; it simply was. In their view, karma was the law of cause and effect—every action has a reaction. According to the venerable Mahasi Sayadaw, "Karma is the result of our own past actions and present doings. We ourselves are responsible for our own happiness and misery—in other words, we create our own heaven and our own hell. We are the architects of our own fate."

The Karma Cleanse taps into the ancient teachings of Ayurveda, the foundation of all Eastern medicine, to give us a taste of the sattvic lifestyle—the middle path of balance, awareness and simplicity that is the ideal of Ayurvedic philosophy. Its practitioners take a unique look at health and disease and create wellness programs tailored to an individual's body type—nutrition, lifestyle and immediate environmental influences are all taken into account. On the nutrition front, they believe that proper digestion is the corner-stone of good health. So one aspect of Ayurveda looks at whether we're eating the right food for our constitutional body type, or dosha. Because we also "digest" what we take in through our mind and our five senses, another tenet of Ayurveda is the belief that everything we think, hear, see, feel and smell also has a profound effect on our body, mind and spirit.

Identify Your Dosha

According to Ayurveda, each of us is born with our own energy blueprint—a combination of the three doshas (Vata, Pitta and Kapha) that governs our physical and emotional health. Deter-mining our dominant dosha, or doshas, gives us insight into the food or lifestyle choices that can keep our body, mind and spirit in balance. People whose primary dosha is Vata (ether/air) bene-fit from foods that are warm, heavy and oily. Those with Pitta (fire) as their dominant dosha benefit from cooling foods. And Kapha (water/earth) types benefit from stimulating, light, dry foods.

The chart on page 116 describes the characteristics of the three doshas. To help you choose from the spice and oil combinations in the recipe and activity sections later in this chapter, review the list to determine what your primary dosha is, or take a quiz at one of the following websites:

* www.ayurveda.com

* www.ayurveda-md.com

* www.eattasteheal.com

For a more thorough analysis of your body type and imbal-ances you may be experiencing, see a licensed Ayurvedic practi-tioner.

Dosha	Sample Characteristics
Vata (ether/air)	Creative; artistic; ethereal; sometimes ungrounded; changeable moods; irregular routine; quick to learn (and forget); thin, tall frame; small facial features; dull complexion; long neck and fingers; dry skin; frequently constipated; fickle appetite; typically has a hard time gaining weight; light sleeper; often feels cold
Pitta (fire)	Sharp; a leader; motivated doer; organized; focused; assertive; obsessive; competitive; stubborn; medium frame; intense eyes; sharp nose; rosy complexion; combination skin that's prone to rashes; thin hair; medium-length neck and fingers; consistent, strong appetite; loose stools; often feels hot
Kapha (water/earth)	Grounded; relaxed; loyal; consistent; likes structure; slow-paced; prone to depression; slow to anger; solid, stocky build; large facial features; thick, wavy hair; oily, moist skin; pale complexion; short neck and fingers; gains weight easily; heavy sleeper; light appetite; slow digestion and elimination; often feels cool

Unlike the meals for the other cleanses in this book, most meals in the Karma Cleanse are cooked "kitchari": a filling combination of legumes, whole grains, spices and vegetables that gives the body protein, good fats and carbohydrates, and a variety of vitamins and minerals. It's easy to digest and helps normalize digestion and absorption of nutrients.

The base of each kitchari recipe is tridoshic, which means it's suitable for Vatas, Pittas and Kaphas, but I include different vegetable and spice blends to add to those bases that are tailored to individual doshas. Once you have an idea of your primary dosha, you'll be able to determine what veggie and spice variation might be best for your body type. I break from strict Ayurvedic tradition and include green juices, sprouts, cooked greens and raw salad in the daily menu to further alkalize the system, help flush the intestines, and add variety and nutrients to the diet.

EATING TO NURTURE THE BODY AND SOUL

Today we often eat quickly, on the run, and at times that differ from one day to the next. A fast eating pace, combined with eating in an tense state, affects our ability to digest, still our minds, and receive the healing power of food with gratitude. Try taking a page out of the rishis' handbook and dine Ayurveda style:

- Eat at the proper times—early in the morning, when the sun is at its highest point (between noon and 2 PM), and before it gets dark (around 5 or 6 PM). Enjoy your main meal when the sun is at its highest point in the sky and eat lighter meals at the start and end of the day. Getting into a routine of eating at the same times each day will aid in digestion.

- Dine in a calm, relaxed mental state. Savor each mouthful. Take several breaths between each forkful.

- Think of your food as an offering to your spirit and a gift from Mother Earth. Cook with loving intent, and pause to reflect and give thanks for the bountiful blessings on your plate before you eat.

- Eat a modest amount of food. The goal is to nourish your body and spirit, rather than trying to feel instantly full.

When to Do the Cleanse

I recommend the Karma Cleanse for people who are thin or weak and for people who want to cleanse during the colder months of the year. It's not for individuals whose primary interest is losing weight. It's ideal when someone is feeling out of balance or their appetite is poor. If someone's feeling disconnected from self or spirit, it rejuvenates the soul. If you're ready to clear your body of foods that adversely affect your health and clear your mind of old baggage and move forward with a fresh perspective, give the Karma Cleanse a try. You can do this cleanse twice each year.

What You'll See and Feel

You'll experience the joy and pleasure of simple, healthy, natural foods. You'll notice a youthful glow and a relaxing of the lines on the skin of your face. You'll gain a sense of calmness, heightened awareness, and a realization that your body is the temple of your spirit.

ABBIE'S TESTIMONIAL

Embarking on a kitchari cleanse and discovering Ayurvedic medicine was such a profound experience for me. Here's what my life was like before the cleanse:

I'd been an athlete my entire life—from the time I was 7, I was competing on the soccer field. When I wasn't playing soccer, I was training, running, hiking, ice-skating, biking, swimming, or using in-line skates. I played soccer in state championships, national championships, and matches overseas and ultimately was offered soccer scholarships to play at universities across the country. In the end, I chose to attend University of Southern California, Los Angeles.

During spring training, I injured my ankle for the second time, and I knew I wouldn't play again. It felt as if the rug was pulled from under me. I couldn't walk well for roughly 6 months, and I realized I'd have to figure out how to develop other parts of myself I'd never connected with up to that point in my life.

Considering that my scholarship was offered to another healthy player, I decided to attend community college to figure out what I should be in life. With a full-time school schedule, I worked full-time and was burning the candle at both ends while I figured out my next move. At the same time, I ate as if I were still in training: lots of pastas and complex carbohydrates, not a lot of vegetables or other good stuff. I had an irregular and imbalanced diet and I could feel my body changing. The combination of diet and lifestyle ended up taking its toll. I became very ill and was diagnosed with mononucleosis.

At that point, I never imagined how big the silver lining was around the storm cloud that apparently had descended over me, and how much this transition was going to change my life.

After hearing my physician say that I'd be sick for at least a month, if not longer, I said to myself, Forget this. I'm going to figure out how to be well on my own. *I was introduced to a book called* Alternative Medicine: The Definitive Guide, *by Burton Goldberg. I looked up* mononucleosis *to see what the book had to say. The book offered information on different herbal recommendations I could take and combinations of alternative therapies I could pursue, so I gave it a go. During that time I went to see an Ayurvedic practitioner, who recommended I try a kitchari cleanse. I had never done a cleanse before, and I wasn't sure I wanted to try one—particularly when I wasn't feeling well—so I decided to wait.*

After a couple of weeks on the herbs, I felt fantastic. I went back for follow-up blood work and the results came back negative for mononucleosis. I had all the proof I needed to know that alternative medicine had incredible power to heal the body. If the herbs and lifestyle modifications worked so well, I figured there might be something to trying a kitchari cleanse.

I embarked on a 15-day kitchari cleanse, tailored to my unique physical needs. Two or three times a day, I ate a meal of mung daal, basmati rice, vegetables and spices. The first day seemed to go okay, the second day was a bit harder, and the third day was the most difficult. My body ached, and I was a little light-headed and tired.

The most difficult part of the cleanse for me was learning how to incorporate a daily routine into my life: rising with the sun, eating when the sun was at its highest point in the sky during the day, eating 2 hours before bed, and going to bed early. I also took a triphala tea, which is a bowel tonic, before bed, to assist with elimination. Before I showered each morning, I would dry-brush my body, with each stroke going toward my heart (to stimulate the lymph and circulatory systems), before massaging in coconut oil.

Once I reached day 4, everything became easier. The detox symptoms subsided and I started to feel the upside of cleansing and honoring a regular daily routine. I was euphoric and had an incredible sustained level of energy. I discovered I needed smaller portions of food to feel energized. My skin was glowing, my eyes were clear and bright, and my body felt at ease.

Eating the same thing for 15 days was quite a discipline. So to keep it interesting, I'd change up the beans, vegetables or spices each day. I'd also drink shots of wheatgrass and/or include some lightly steamed vegetables with my kitchari meals.

During the cleansing process, I noticed I wanted to slow down. As I started to feel more conscious and aware, my senses became more acute. My biorhythms became more in tune with nature; I felt more grounded and connected to my environment.

Ultimately, after learning how embarking on a cleanse nurtured my mind, body and spirit, I began studying Eastern healing modalities. What started as an exercise in healing my own body became my life path of helping others develop a deeper connection to themselves in relationship to the outside world. Today I have become an Ayurvedic practitioner as a guide to assisting others with their healing.

To this day, I cleanse seasonally, and often on Sundays, to clear my body and mind, honor the natural rhythms of Mother Earth, and reconnect with self and the energy of all that surrounds. For me, cleans-

ing has become a ritual to offer gratitude for the preciousness of human life and all we have to be thankful for.

CLEANSE AT A GLANCE

Rise with the sun

On waking: Hot Lemon Water (see recipe page 33)

Through the day: Ginger, licorice, tulsi tea or Juice of Amrit

Breakfast: Kitchari with vegetables

Lunch (when the sun is at its highest, between noon and 2 PM): Kitchari with vegetables

Snack (optional): Chakra Salad with Lemon Dressing

Dinner (before dark): Kitchari with vegetables

Before bed (to aid in elimination): Triphala tea

Hit the sack by 10 PM.

Special Equipment

✳ Juicer
✳ Fine sieve

RECIPES

NOTE: Triphala powder, wheatgrass shots and essential oils are available at health-food stores. Ghee and kombu are available at Asian markets.

JUICE OF AMRIT

Makes 1 serving

Ayurvedic myth tells the tale of the god Amrit, who created a potion bringing long, healthy lives to those who drank it. His recipe has been lost, but I think the megadose of chlorophyll, enzymes and vitamins in this juice could mimic the fabled brew. Including a raw juice in a kitchari cleanse is unconventional, but some of my colleagues and I craved fresh greens when we did a kitchari cleanse, so I've included it here.

1/2 head celery (4–5 stalks)
1/2 cucumber
1/2 apple, cored
7 chard leaves, beet greens or kale
2 cups pea sprouts or sprouts of your choice
One 1-inch piece fresh ginger, peeled
2 tablespoons fresh lemon

Directions: Chop the first 4 ingredients into pieces small enough to fit into the feed tube of your juicer. Juice each of the ingredients, starting with the celery and ending with the cucumber and apple to ensure that you get every drop of juice from the chard, sprouts and ginger. Pour into a glass and add lemon juice and enough water to bring the juice up to 16 ounces. Stir and enjoy.

CHAKRA SALAD WITH LEMON DRESSING

Makes 2 servings

I can't imagine going a week without eating a crunchy salad, so I'm putting a modern twist on a kitchari cleanse by including a recipe for one of my favorites. The combination of the crunchy lettuce and jicama, bitter endive, peppery arugula, creamy avocado and tart dressing wakes up your taste buds! And studies show that cilantro is effective at pulling heavy metals out of the body.

Salad
1/4 head romaine lettuce, chopped into bite-sized pieces
1/4 cup fennel, chopped into bite-sized pieces
1 medium tomato, chopped into bite-sized pieces
1 cup sprouts of your choice
1 handful baby arugula
1/4 avocado, peeled, seeded and chopped into small dice
1/4 cup jicama, peeled and chopped into small dice
1 tablespoon cilantro, chopped

Directions: Mix the romaine, endive, tomato, sprouts, arugula, avocado, jicama and cilantro together in a large bowl. Pour dressing over salad and toss well. Transfer to a plate or eat it right out of the bowl!

DRESSING

1 tablespoon flax oil
4 teaspoons fresh lemon juice
1/4 teaspoon garlic, minced
Pinch of Himalayan or Celtic sea salt

Directions: Whisk ingredients together in a bowl.

THE MIRACLES OF GHEE

Ghee is a type of clarified butter used in Ayurveda to stimulate assimilation of vitamins A, E, D, and K and absorption of other nutrients. The clarification process removes the saturated fats. Ghee is believed to nourish all tissues in the body, increase flexibility and improve immunity. Used in moderation, it's tridoshic, but it's especially soothing to Vata and Pitta. Ghee can be purchased at Asian markets and health-food stores, or you can try the following recipe from Debra Riordan, clinical Ayurvedic specialist and one of my teachers at the College of Ayurveda, in Grass Valley, California, if you'd like to make your own.

1 calm, meditative cook
1 pound unsalted organic butter
1 mason jar
1 heavy stainless-steel pan
Serving spoon for skimming
2 plates for skimmed solids
Fine sieve, or 2 sheets cheesecloth, folded in half

Directions: Sterilize jar and serving spoon in boiling water for 2 to 3 minutes and set aside to dry. The jar must be completely clean and dry before use. Heat the butter gently in a saucepan on a medium-low setting, stirring continuously. Use the serving spoon to skim off the foam onto plates. Continue skimming and stirring for 15 to 25 minutes. When the ghee starts to smell like buttered popcorn and the color turns a golden color, immediately remove the pan from the burner. Stir one last time and let the ghee settle for 20 to 25 minutes. Pour the ghee into the jar through the sieve or cheesecloth. Ghee can be stored, refrigerated, for 1 month.

KITCHARI BASES

The following kitchari recipes put a modern spin on a traditional kitchari cleanse with the addition of steamed vegetables. All three kitchari bases are tridoshic, meaning they're suitable for Vatas, Pittas and Kaphas. You tailor the recipes to your dominant dosha with the vegetables and spices you add to the base. All three kitchari bases should be cooked slowly, with care taken not to overcook the grains and legumes. It's a 5-day cleanse, so consider trying more than one of the kitchari bases to keep your palate interested.

Millet Kitchari

Makes 5 servings

2 cups millet
7½ cups purified water
½ teaspoon Himalayan or Celtic sea salt
½ cup dried garbanzo beans, soaked overnight
One 1-inch strip kombu
1 tablespoon ghee, melted
1 teaspoon cumin
1 teaspoon coriander
Generous pinch of turmeric
1 teaspoon fennel seed
Optional: splash of umeboshi vinegar

Directions: Place millet in a fine sieve and rinse well to clean. Add millet to a 4-quart pot and toast over high heat, stirring continuously, until the water has evaporated and the millet begins to lightly change color and emit a gentle aroma. Add 3½ cups water and bring to a boil. Cover and let simmer over low heat for about 30 minutes, until water is evaporated. In a separate pot, add the soaked garbanzo beans and the remaining 4 cups of water. Bring to a boil, reduce heat, and simmer for 45 minutes. When beans are tender and millet is finished cooking, transfer both to large bowl, add remaining ingredients and your choice of dosha-specific herbs or spices (see pages 130–131), and mix to blend. Plate up a 1-cup serving of the kitchari base and top with ½ cup dosha-specific steamed vegetables (see pages 128–130). For extra flavor, add additional cumin or coriander, if desired, and optional splash of umeboshi vinegar to your bowl. (Use it sparingly; it's very salty.)

Quinoa Kitchari

Makes 5 servings

8 cups purified water
2 cups quinoa
½ cup dried French lentils, soaked overnight
½ cup sprouts of your choice
1 tablespoon cilantro, chopped
2 tablespoons flax or olive oil
½ teaspoon Himalayan or Celtic sea salt
1 teaspoon cumin
1 teaspoon coriander
Generous pinch of turmeric
1 teaspoon fennel seeds

Directions: Bring 4 cups of water to a boil in a medium pot. Add quinoa, reduce heat, cover, and simmer for 20 minutes or until the water has been absorbed. In a separate pot, pour in the soaked lentils and the remaining 4 cups of water. Bring to a boil, reduce heat, and simmer for 20 minutes. Transfer quinoa and lentils to a large mixing bowl, add the remaining ingredients and your choice of dosha-specific herbs or spices (see pages 130–131), and mix to combine. Plate up a 1-cup serving of the kitchari base, top with ½ cup of dosha-specific steamed vegetables (see pages 128–130), and enjoy!

Brown Rice Kitchari

Makes 5 servings

2 cups brown rice
8 cups purified water
½ cup mung beans, soaked overnight
One 1-inch strip kombu
1 tablespoon ghee
½ teaspoon Himalayan or Celtic sea salt
1 teaspoon cumin, or more to taste
1 teaspoon ground coriander, or more to taste
Generous pinch of turmeric
1 teaspoon fennel seed

Directions: Add rice and 4 cups of water to a 4-quart pot. Bring to boil. Reduce heat, cover tightly and simmer for 45 minutes. In a separate pot bring mung beans, and the remaining 4 cups of water and kombu to a boil. Cover with a tight-fitting lid, reduce heat and simmer for 15 to 20 minutes. Turn off heat and let sit, uncovered, for 10 minutes. Transfer rice and mung bean mixture to a large mixing bowl, take out kombu and set aside, add the remaining ingredients and your choice of dosha-specific herbs or spices (see pages 130–131), and mix to combine. Plate up a 1-cup serving of the kitchari base, top with ½ cup of dosha-specific steamed vegetables (see pages 128–130), and enjoy!

Steamed Vegetables, by Dosha

Add ½ cup of raw or lightly steamed veggies to each portion of kitchari. If the veggies are cooked, duration of steaming will vary by vegetable. Try changing vegetables day to day—or even meal to meal—to add some variety to your diet.

Vata Veggies
Vata is balanced by foods that are sweet, salty and sour. Cooked vegetables are best.

Avocados
Beets
Carrots
Leeks
Mustard greens
Onions
Acorn squash
Sweet potatoes
Tomatoes
Water chestnuts
Artichoke
Asparagus
Green leafy vegetables
Arugula
Parsnip
Kabocha squash

Pitta Veggies
Sweet, bitter and astringent foods bring Pitta back into balance. Pitta vegetables can be eaten raw in the summer and steamed in the colder months. Pittas should beware of hot chilies, mustard greens, radishes and raw onions, which are hot and pungent.

Sprouts
Lettuce
Artichoke
Asparagus
Broccoli
Cabbage
Cauliflower
Green bell peppers
Peas
Squash
Cucumbers
Watercress
Pumpkin
Seaweed
Kale and other leafy greens

Kapha Veggies

Kaphas need pungent, bitter and astringent food to stimulate their systems.

Sprouts
Green beans
Asparagus
Cabbage
Brussels sprouts
Celery
Carrots
Broccoli
Chilies
Cilantro
Leafy greens
Radishes
Parsley

Hot peppers
Artichokes
Potatoes
Parsley
Seaweed
Spinach
Rutabaga

Herb and Spice Combinations, by Dosha

Vata Spices
To balance Vatas, use a moderate amount of spice and avoid food that's very hot or bland. (Choose 1 or 2.)

1 tablespoon chopped basil
½ teaspoon dill
⅛ teaspoon cinnamon
⅛ teaspoons hing
⅛ teaspoon anise

Pitta Spices
Pittas need cooling, soothing spice options. (Choose one or experiment with a combination of the following.)

1 tablespoon shredded coconut
1 tablespoon chopped cilantro
1 tablespoon chopped dill
1 tablespoon chopped mint
1 tablespoon fresh lime juice

Kapha Spices
Kaphas are balanced by stimulating spices. (Choose 1 or 2; some of these are hot spices, so add them sparingly.)

1 tablespoon chopped basil
1 tablespoon chopped marjoram or oregano
1/8 teaspoon cayenne
1/8 tablespoon black pepper
1 teaspoon minced fresh ginger
1 teaspoon mustard seeds
1/8 teaspoon hing
1/2 teaspoon minced chili pepper
1/8 teaspoon red pepper flakes

TRIPHALA TEA

Makes 1 serving

To keep your bowels moving during a kitchari cleanse, drink a cup of triphala tea 30 minutes before bedtime. Its gentle laxative effect helps eliminate excess doshas and toxins from the body and keeps the digestion and excretory systems functioning smoothly. Powdered triphala is available at health-food stores.

1/4 teaspoon–1 teaspoon powdered triphala (Vatas and Kaphas will
   need more triphala than Pittas will)
1 cup hot purified water

Directions: Bring water to a boil and transfer to a cup or mug. Stir in the triphala and allow to steep for 10 minutes, until all the powder settles. Drink. If there is too much of a laxative effect, decrease the dosage.

Cleanse-Boosting Activities

Rub It In

Before you bathe, massage your entire body with the oil suited to your primary dosha (sesame oil for Vata, coconut oil for Pitta and almond oil for Kapha). Rub the oil into your skin in broad, gentle strokes, working in the direction of your heart. After the oil is absorbed, take a hot bath or shower to help sweat toxins out of your body—a steam or sauna is an even better option, if that's available. Doing this each day stimulates circulation, draws toxins out of the tissues and organs, and speeds up the elimination of wastes. It's also nourishing and balancing for the entire body-mind.

If you'd like a scented oil, try adding a few drops of essential oil—tailored to your dominant dosha—to 4 ounces of the base oil. Here's a breakdown of some essential oils by dosha:

* Vata: choose a warming scent, such as basil, sandalwood or ginger.

* Pitta: choose a cooling and calming fragrance, such as lavender, rose or jasmine.

* Kapha: choose a scent that's stimulating, such as eucalyptus, cinnamon or orange oil.

Gimme an "Om"

Chakra is a Sanskrit word meaning "wheel," and it refers to the seven energy centers that run along our spine. Each chakra has a particular focus or function but, collectively, they regulate the flow of energy throughout our bodies. Our thoughts, feelings and perceptions all determine whether these "energy valves" are open or closed. When a chakra is closed or stressed, it isn't able to direct the appropriate energy into the body, and we ultimately experience the physical symptoms of that pipeline begin to cut off. In this exercise, we chant bija mantras to clear out stuck energy and get those chakra wheels spinning so that we can achieve a greater sense of balance and harmony (see page 134 for more on bija mantras).

To get started, sit or lie down in a comfortable position. I enjoy sitting in the cross-legged lotus position on a cushion or rug. You'll be chanting the bija mantras for each chakra, starting with the bija for the first chakra, moving to the bija for the second chakra, and so on, until you reach the silent bija for the seventh chakra at the crown of your head.

✳ Take a few deep, cleansing breaths.

✳ After a deep inhale, chant the bija *lam* (pronounced "lahm") for 4 seconds.

✳ Inhale for a count of 4 seconds and then chant the second chakra bija, *vam* (pronounced "vahm"), for 4 seconds.

✳ Proceed up the spine, alternating 4-second inhalations with 4-second chants of the bija for each chakra (see table below for bijas).

✳ At the seventh chakra, simply sit in meditative silence, focusing on the crown chakra atop your head.

✳ Repeat for 5 minutes. As you get more comfortable with the process and begin feeling the positive shift of energy in your body, you may find you want to extend this practice to 10, 15 or more minutes each day.

Chakra	Location	Bija Mantra
First	Base of the spine	Lam ("lahm")
Second	Below the navel	Vam ("vahm")
Third	Just below the rib cage	Ram ("rahm")
Fourth	Center of the chest	Yam ("yahm")
Fifth	Throat	Hum ("hoom")
Sixth	Center of the brow	Om ("ohm")
Seventh	Just above the head	(Silence)

WHAT'S A BIJA MANTRA?

Bija mantras, or seed mantras, are one-word syllables that the rishis described as eternal, conscious, living sounds. Each bija sound has its own transformative power and represents an elemental force of energy in the chakras. Chanting the different seed sounds of each chakra in succession is a great way to clear blocked energy and get those chakras shining at the start of your day!

Chanting bija mantras is also believed to help integrate the right and left sides of our brains—which usually operate in different modes, on different wavelengths. Combined with a quiet, meditative state, the rhythmic sounds of the bija mantras sync up both sides of the brain. When this happens, we can achieve a greater sense of clarity and heightened awareness—we can visualize more easily, better understand our emotions, tap deeper in our creativity and see solutions to situations more clearly.

Start Up Your Sun Salutations

Yoga is an ideal activity for the Karma Cleanse because yoga and Ayurveda have a long history together as complementary ways of healing the body and bringing us into harmony with nature. In Sanskrit, *yoga* means "to unite," and its goal is to fully integrate the body, mind and spirit by

✳ Maintaining the flexibility and integrity of our joints and spine

✳ Strengthening and stretching the body to balance muscles in relationship to each other

✳ Clearing the body's energy system and regulating energy flow

✳ Stimulating the glandular, nervous, cardiovascular and digestive systems

✳ Cleansing and nourishing the body on every level

✳ Shedding light on behaviors or attitudes that could be holding us in place and keeping us from achieving our highest potential

So check into classes at local yoga studios or recreational centers. Classes in the ashtanga or hatha forms of yoga complement this cleanse best.

THE SUPER SLIM-DOWN
CLEANSE (7 DAYS)

The Super Slim-Down Cleanse is not a fad or crash diet; it's a catalyst for change in which you take a leap into being one with your body and staying committed to a healthier path. Will you lose weight? Yes, but most important, you won't be starving, and you'll look and feel so much better. If all goes as planned, you'll have a whole new perspective on what you choose to eat—one that will last into the future. So look at this week as a celebration! You're about to embark on a journey into a whole new way of being.

That's because the Super Slim-Down is the perfect prescription for weaning yourself off the standard American diet (SAD), eliminating cravings for sugar, meat, alcohol, caffeine and junk food. It's a nutritional cleanse that leaves you feeling satisfied because it's delivering what your body is *really* craving. It boosts your body's ability to heal when your system is taxed, gets you back into balance, and lifts you out of any mental fog so you can feel recharged and revitalized.

I went back to the kitchen and whipped up recipes that add a little extra joy. There are a number of things that give this cleanse an added punch: I've included a morning smoothie packed with protein, fiber and antioxidants; pineapple for its useful digestive enzymes and vitamins; and the ancient Mayan chia seed for sustained energy, fiber and essential fatty acids. I've also built in a quick way to grow your own low-cost, super-protein sprouts.

I've been perfecting this cleanse over the last several years with my clients, and the feedback has been great. Everyone loves the new recipes, and they're losing weight and keeping it off by building them into their ongoing meal plans! That's because the Super Slim-Down helps you break your addictions to poor food choices, building your confidence and elevating your mood while it detoxifies and rejuvenates. It's almost impossible not to want to eat differently after doing this cleanse!

If your experience is similar to my clients' experiences, this week will dramatically alter what you crave and give you 20/20 hindsight into how you felt when you weren't eating this way. To help you stay on the path and incorporate what you've learned into your daily routine, I recommend reading the Breaking the Cleanse section (page 209) to get a handle on the big picture.

I want hear how you're doing, so stay in touch and email me at adina@adinaniemerow.com. Share your stories, celebrate your successes, and ask me questions. I'll reply and choose stories and questions to post on my website so other cleansers can join the dialogue and learn more about the cleanse experience.

P.S. If you decide to do this cleanse for longer than a week, you can build some variety into the daily routine by including soups and juices from the Urban Revitalizer and Green Buzz cleanses.

When to Do the Cleanse

If you want to shed a few pounds but don't want to starve your body. If you're ready to take a week off from alcohol, coffee, bagels, cheese and pastries. If the food you eat on a daily basis is slowing you down and you're looking for an easy introduction into a clean diet. If you've slipped into a routine of having a few glasses of wine or cups of coffee a day.

What You'll See and Feel

With the fog lifted and pounds shed (my clients typically lose 2 to 7 pounds), you might find you're popping out of bed in the morning clear-eyed. The urge for that morning coffee or third glass of wine might be a thing of the past. You'll notice that the foods you were eating before the cleanse were making you feel tired and you'll become aware of just how addictive white bread, sugar, coffee and alcohol are. Day by day you'll see your craving for clean foods grow, and you'll be inspired to think more about where your food comes from and what's in it.

Sprouted beans are what give this cleanse an extra protein punch. While beans are vegetarian, once they sprout, their growth mechanism kicks in and they transform into little enzymatic protein powerhouses! These don't look anything like the bean sprouts you get in dishes at Asian restaurants—they're small and look like a seed with a tail. The great news is, they're the cheapest, easiest-to-digest form of protein out there—so set aside a tiny space in your kitchen to grow your own. It's easy, but they take three days to sprout, so build that time into your menu planning before your start the cleanse. See the Make Room to Grow activity on page 148 for the easy instructions.

DEE AND AVI'S TESTIMONIAL

Dee: *I'm married to a major carnivore who happens to be kick-ass in the kitchen. There isn't a fine meal or down-home comfort food dish he can't whip up to perfection. My taste buds might have been celebrating, but it's been a slippery slope for my body. Actually, over the past* *three years, it's been more like a cliff. Work took over my life; I stopped exercising and fed my body lots of really fattening, empty calories. I was worn out and depressed. When the bottom fell out of the economy a few years ago, Avi's business was hit hard and it caused a lot of stress for us. Several wines, beers or cocktails became part of the daily routine, and we went from being "social smokers" to smoking like chimneys . . .*

Avi: *Speak for yourself!*

Dee: *Oh, please! Bottom line: we'd been punishing our bodies and were looking and feeling like crap—it was affecting our moods, our marriage and our lives. We both finally hit this point where we said* enough.

Avi: *Yeah. Plus, I sail and I've been getting invited onto more and more competitive boats. But my weight was holding me back. To be a bowman on the boats I wanted to race on, I needed to lose thirty pounds.*

Dee: *And to get back into a bikini, I need to lose at least twenty. So we agreed we'd do a cleanse together. I'd tried a liquid cleanse six years ago, but it was tough, and I'd been a lot healthier leading up to it. Plus, I knew we'd both be dealing with alcohol and tobacco withdrawal while we were cleansing, so we needed something easier.*

Avi: *And there was no way I was going to do a cleanse that didn't include solid food. Forget that.*

Dee: *So we talked to Adina and agreed the Super Slim-Down would be the best route to go. We jumped right in and I was amazed. From the first day, I was never hungry—in fact I found I was skipping one of the soups or juices each day because I felt full.*

Avi: *Not me . . . I felt hungry. I wasn't a huge fan of the cold soups and I wanted more solid foods, so I spoke with Adina and she said I could* *have a small piece of fish at lunch. She also said I could substitute small portions of the raw veggie dishes or warm soups from other chapters in the book for the cold soups. Adding a bit of fish and making substitutions were key to my sticking with it, no doubt.*

Dee: *And I was so proud he did! I decided to continue on for a second week, and he agreed to doing a modified version of the cleanse with me. I chalk that up to the fact that this cleanse was relatively gentle and that Adina was flexible in building in the elements Avi needed to stay on track. It wasn't all roses—we both had some detox symptoms: we felt a little flu-ish for the first two or three days; we needed Swiss Kriss tablets to keep the old bowels moving; and we were irritable at the start. Given all we'd been eating, drinking and smoking leading up to this, I wasn't surprised—we were feeling a little raw. What did surprise me is the fact that I'd been talking and talking about giving up smoking leading up to this, and now I've finally done it.*

Avi: *It was strange that neither of us was craving alcohol or cigarettes—maybe it was mind over matter, but we'd made a commitment to doing this and we were going to follow through. Something else I didn't expect—the fast-food commercials I was salivating over at the start of the cleanse are making my stomach turn now . . . that food just doesn't even look good. Now, don't get me wrong—I'm not giving up alcohol, and I'm not saying I'll never eat meat or cheese or breads or pastas or desserts again. I definitely will, and I'll love eating them (although Adina tells me I'll enjoy them less than I did before . . . we'll see). But I'll have them less frequently and I won't be piling up the plate the way I used to. It's interesting to see that smaller portions are enough to fill you up.*

Dee: *Yeah, we're seeing and feeling a difference. In the first week, we lost our bloat and dropped a few pounds—I could definitely see it in* *my face and feel it in my pants. We don't want to lose that, so we've both decided the breakfast smoothie and green juices are permanent fixtures of our daily routine, and we'll be cooking other recipes from the book throughout the week.*

Avi: Absolutely. I didn't do the cleanse totally by the book, and I still felt better and noticed a difference. I actually think doing it that way versus doing a hard-core cleanse helped show me how we can eat this way for the long haul, not just while we're cleansing.

CLEANSE AT A GLANCE

On waking: 1 or 2 cups hot water with lemon juice (at least one teaspoon lemon juice per cup)

7:00 a.m.: Mighty Green Juice (Optional—SOS breakfast cereal, only if you have to add a hot breakfast)*

9:00 a.m.: Electrolyte Shake or Purple Smoothie

11:30 a.m.: Mighty Green Juice

1:00 p.m.: Super Sprout Salad with Sesame Dressing and Roasted Yam Slices

2:30 p.m.: Pine-Avo Watercress Soup

3:30 p.m.: Cha-Cha Chia Shot

4:30 p.m.: Mighty Green Juice

6:30 p.m.: Chilled Creamy Spinach Soup

Bedtime: Take 2 Swiss Kriss tablets or 3 rounded teaspoons Natural Calm (magnesium powder that helps move the bowels)

*I recommend the juice or smoothie for your breakfast option, but some folks need a warm breakfast

Special Equipment

* ✳ High-speed blender
* ✳ Juicer
* ✳ Fine-mesh sieve or nut-milk bag
* ✳ Parchment paper

NOTE: The mung beans need to sprout for three days before they're ready to eat, so build that into your pre-cleanse planning. See the Make Room to Grow activity on page 148 for instructions. I highly recommend making your own nut milk (see page 93), but you can also purchase unsweetened almond milk at health food stores and a growing number of grocery stores. Young coconuts or coconut water (also called coconut juice) have also gone mainstream and can be found in many supermarkets, or you can find them in health food stores and Asian markets. If you choose to buy a young coconut, see page 160 for instructions on how to open it.

RECIPES

MIGHTY GREEN JUICE

Makes 2 servings

This green juice is life force energy in a glass. Chock-full of enzymes and chlorophyll, it will clean your blood and help bring you back into alkaline balance.

1 large cucumber
5 celery stalks
1 small apple, cored
3 kale leaves
3 chard leaves
Optional super food: 2 cups pea or sunflower sprouts
Juice of a lemon, to taste

Directions: Chop the first five ingredients into pieces small enough to fit into the feed tube of your juicer. Juice the ingredients in order to ensure you get every drop of juice from the kale, chard and sprouts (if using). Pour into a glass, stir in the lemon juice, and drink in the power!

OPTIONAL SOS BREAKFAST CEREAL

Makes 1 serving

Buckwheat is really tasty and it's a gluten-free grain, so it's easy to digest. I like the Pocono brand, but if you can't find that, buy buckwheat in bulk and grind in a coffee grinder or blender until fine. Add a few berries and a couple of chopped almonds if you must.

1 cup purified water or almond milk
Pinch of salt
¼ cup buckwheat

Directions: Bring the water and pinch of salt to boil in a small saucepan over high heat. Stir in the buckwheat and return to a boil. Reduce the heat to low and simmer 10 minutes or until thickened to taste, stirring frequently.

ELECTROLYTE SHAKE

Makes 2 servings

Almonds are rich in calcium, iron and phosphorus. I recommend buying raw almonds from the farmers' market since almonds at grocery stores have been pasteurized, killing their enzymes. For variety, you can experiment by substituting hazelnuts, pumpkin-seeds or Brazil nuts for the almonds.

¼ cup raw almonds, soaked overnight and then drained
3 cups coconut water or purified water
1 cup purified water
Optional: pinch of cinnamon or vanilla bean seeds

Directions: Process the first 3 ingredients in a blender until smooth, then strain through a fine sieve or nut-milk bag. Rinse the blender. Pour the mixture back into blender with the optional ingredient (if using) and blend to incorporate. Pour half the milk into a glass and enjoy. The remaining milk will keep for 2 days in the refrigerator.

PURPLE SMOOTHIE

Makes 1 serving

This smoothie is habit-forming. It will jump-start your morning and make you feel good from head to toe. You can use raspberries or strawberries, but I choose blueberries for their brain-enhancing nutrients. Be sure to choose a non-whey, non-soy-based protein powder to keep the smoothie easy to digest—I love the berry-flavored Vega Complete Whole Food Health Optimizer.

1 cup purified water
1 cup coconut water (I like Amy & Brian's All Natural coconut juice)
1/4 cup berries
1 to 2 scoops of protein powder
2 Brazil nuts
Optional: scoop of green powder of your choice (I use Progreens)

Directions: Place all ingredients in a blender and blend until smooth. Pour into a glass and sip the liquid bliss!

SUPER SPROUT SALAD WITH CREAMY SESAME DRESSING AND ROASTED YAM SLICES

Makes 2 servings

This fresh, filling and crunchy salad will keep your taste buds happy and your tummy satisfied. The home-grown sprouts are packed with lo-cal, easy-to-digest protein—pure power for the body. And once you taste the thinly sliced and roasted yams, they'll be your new best friend.

2 small yams (not quite 1 pound)
1 head romaine lettuce, shredded
1/2 cabbage, shredded
2 tablespoons chopped cilantro
1 cup sunflower sprouts
1 cucumber, diced small
1 cup sprouted mung beans (see page 149)
2 teaspoons black (or white) sesame seeds
Creamy Sesame Dressing (see recipe below)

Directions: To roast the yams, preheat the oven to 400°F. Wash the yams and cut them into thin slices. Line a cooking sheet with lightly oiled parchment paper. Arrange the yam slices in a single layer on the sheet and roast for 15 minutes, or until crisp. Remove and set aside to cool. The roasted yam slices can be stored in an airtight container for several days.

Toss the remaining ingredients in a large bowl. Serve on plates, top with several roasted yam slices, drizzle with sesame dressing, and enjoy!

CREAMY SESAME DRESSING

4 tablespoons extra virgin olive oil
3 tablespoons fresh lemon juice
1½ teaspoons Bragg Liquid Aminos
1 teaspoon ume plum vinegar
1 teaspoon sesame seeds
Option: 1 teaspoon raw honey

Directions: Place all ingredients in a blender or mini food processor and mix well. This recipe makes enough for 2 servings, so keep extra dressing chilled in the refrigerator until you're ready to use it.

PINE-AVO WATERCRESS SOUP

Makes 1 serving

I have been captivated with pineapples this year. The combination of the sweet pineapple, tart greens, and zippy ginger and jalapeño will light up your palate while the enzymes, bromelin and vitamin C in the pineapple light up your body! This yummy recipe was concocted by one of my cleansers, Lori Hunter. Not into pineapple? No problem, just substitute cucumber.

2 cups fresh pineapple chunks
2 tablespoons chopped watercress or arugula
1 tablespoon peeled and minced gingerroot
1 cup water
½ avocado
1 tablespoon seeded, finely chopped jalapeno
1 teaspoon chopped mint

Directions: Add all the ingredients to your blender and puree until smooth.

CHA-CHA CHIA SHOT

Makes 1 serving

This shot of vital nourishment will give you a jolt of omega-3 fatty acids, protein, antioxidants and fiber. It's been known to scare off hunger, so you can drink this at other times during the day, or add it to soups or smoothies, if you feel like your tank needs a top-off.

2 teaspoons chia seeds
¼ cup coconut water

Directions: Soak the chia seeds in coconut water overnight in the refrigerator. Pour into a shot glass and enjoy.

CHILLED CREAMY SPINACH SOUP

Makes 1 serving

This soup is my green dream machine: it's easy to make and flat-out tastes great. I like to spike mine with a ton of hot sauce. I'm a big fan of cilantro, but you can experiment with other herbs as well—if you choose a strong herb such as thyme, tarragon or marjoram, you'll just need a little pinch.

2 cups fresh spinach
1 cup water
½ avocado
1 celery stalk, chopped
2 tablespoons fresh lemon juice
1 tablespoon fresh chopped cilantro
1 teaspoon Bragg Liquid Aminos
A dash or two of hot sauce (or load it up with hot sauce like I do!)

Directions: Put all the ingredients into a blender and puree until smooth.

DRINK UP!

Think you've had enough water? Chances are you haven't had enough. Staying well hydrated is critical to flushing toxins from the body as you cleanse. So toss some thinly sliced cucumber into your water or squeeze in some lemon juice, and keep sipping away!

Cleanse-Boosting Activities

Make Room to Grow

The time of the sprout has come, and I'm spreading the word! I'm always searching for healthy alternative sources of eco-friendly, sustainably grown protein other than nuts, seeds and soy, and I've discovered the perfect solution. Research done at Purdue University shows that sprouted beans contain extraordinary levels of good-quality protein. For example, 25 percent of the calories in mung bean sprouts come from protein—that's a greater percentage than the calories from protein found in a T-bone steak! And they contain none of the fat, cholesterol, antibiotics or hormones found in most meat products today. Even more exciting, sprouted foods give us the most digestible, concentrated source of vitamins, minerals, enzymes and amino acids on the planet. I've been testing these little power-houses and they're a tasty and satisfying delicacy. I honestly feel more energized after eating a little bowl of these jewels.

So, create your own sprout "garden" in your kitchen. It takes very little space to grow economical, easy-to-digest proteins that you can use both during the cleanse and after the cleanse to replace meat in recipes you make. The following instructions are for mung bean sprouts, but you could also sprout peas, lentils, garbanzo beans, adzuki beans—the possibilities are endless!

Sprouting Instructions

✳ Rinse 1 cup of mung beans in a fine mesh colander and pick through them to remove any pebbles.

✳ Fill a large bowl with 6 cups of purified water and add the rinsed, picked beans.

✳ Soak the beans for 24 hours, drain them through a fine mesh colander, and rinse thoroughly.

✳ Rinse out the bowl you soaked the beans in and set the strainer filled with beans over the bowl so that the beans can continue draining. Set aside to let the sprouting process start.

✳ Rinse the beans twice a day and place the colander filled with mung beans back over the rinsed bowl to continue draining.

✳ After 2 days, once you see the beans growing tails, they're ready to add into the recipes! Rinse a final time and drain well.

✳ Well-drained beans can be refrigerated in a tightly sealed glass container that's lined with paper towels for up to 5 days.

Sweat Your Prayers

Every Sunday morning in Sausalito, California, people come from all over the greater San Francisco Bay Area to listen to great DJs, shake their booty and sweat their prayers in Gabrielle Roth's 5Rhythms dance program. It's a simple, powerful moving meditation that anyone—of any age, size or physical ability—can practice. There are no steps to follow; there's no choreography to learn or way to do it wrong. The only requirements are a body that's still breathing, a heart that's still beating and a mind that's still curious!

"To sweat is to pray, to make an offering of your innermost self. Sweat is holy water, prayer beads, pearls of liquid that release your past. Sweat is an ancient and universal form of self-healing, whether done in the gym, the sauna or the sweat lodge. I do it on the dance floor. The more you dance, the more you sweat. The more you sweat, the more you pray. The more you pray, the closer you come to ecstasy."
—GABRIELLE ROTH

Just like light, sound or ocean waves, a dancing body when moving freely passes through five distinct rhythmic patterns. These patterns continuously repeat themselves in a wave of motion. The tenets of Roth's 5Rhythms are:

✳ **Flowing**—the fluid, continuous, grounded glide of our own movements

✳ **Staccato**—the percussive, pulsing beat that shapes us a thousand different ways

✳ **Chaos**—the rhythm of letting go, releasing into the catalytic wildness of our dance that can never be planned or repeated

✳ **Lyrical**—the rhythm of trance, where the weight of self-consciousness dissolves, where we lighten up and disappear into our own uniqueness

✳ **Stillness**—the quiet emptiness, where gentle movements rise and fall, start and end, in a field of silence

You don't need to live in the Bay Area to experience this amazing meditation. Check out 5Rhythms online to see what resources are available to help you sweat your prayers wherever you live, and let the music shift your vibration!

Keep Company

It's challenging to do a cleanse when friends and family are feasting around you. Rather than feeling isolated while you eat, choose recipes from this book and prepare a meal for all of you. No need to tell them in advance that they'll be enjoying delicious vegetarian food and clean tea cocktails—seeing (and eating) is believing! Set the mood for a special meal—lay a beautiful table, light candles, and put on some great tunes. You'll have the pleasure of enjoying a great evening with loved ones while sticking to your commitment to cleanse. Who knows . . . once you tell them the recipes were from your cleanse, you may have a few recruits!

If your cleansing experience is like that of many Super Cleansers, you'll finish the cleanse on a high. You'll believe in the rejuvenating power of clean, balanced and nutritious food; and you'll want to eat differently on an ongoing basis. You can eat clean and keep company after the cleanse by incorporating recipes from this book into your daily or weekly routines. Going to a dinner party? Offer to bring a dish along to contribute to the gathering. Hosting a party? Create a spread from my recipes. In addition to the recipes from this chapter, scan the Laughing Buddha, "Some Like It Raw" and Mexican Fiesta chapters for great crowd-pleasing recipes.

You don't need to tell people you've created delicious, life-giving foods. The proof is in the pudding (or the soup, salad or entrée)! Once they get a taste, they'll be back for more!

THE URBAN REVITALIZER CLEANSE (5 DAYS)

Does the world around you seem to be made of concrete and asphalt? Are skyscrapers dwarfing all of the trees? Can you remember the last time you watched the moon rise or sun set, or listened to birds sing? Is the pace of city life wearing you down?

I've lived in big cities for most of my life, from New York to L.A. to San Francisco, so I know what it's like to get caught up in the rush and the intensity. Don't get me wrong . . . I love a lot of things about city living. But always being on the go can have a domino effect.

Those of us living in urban environments are often under more stress then those living elsewhere, because of fast-paced activities and harmful environmental factors. And life on the run can get chaotic—we get too rushed to eat healthy food, too busy to relax and take time to reflect or care for ourselves, too stressed to get the sleep we need. It all adds up and takes a toll on the body.

When we're stressed out, we sometimes cope in ways that make the situation even worse, such as eating fast food, smoking or drinking more, or not exercising because we feel so exhausted. We'll grab a quick shot of espresso or chocolate bar just to keep ourselves going. Problem is, that stuff won't do the trick after a while—and, frankly, it only adds to the stress the body is under.

We have to be able to return to a relaxed, pre-stress state—if we don't, our body becomes overworked and our energy resources are depleted. In addition, acid levels in the body rise and the digestive and immune systems are ultimately compromised. This in turn opens us up to a host of physical and emotional ailments. Researchers estimate that as many as 75% to 90% of all visits to a physician's office are linked to stress-related problems.

ARE YOU STRESSED OUT?

The following physical and emotional symptoms may be signs that you're experiencing levels of stress that could ultimately lead to more serious health problems:

- Exhaustion and ongoing fatigue

- Feeling mentally foggy

- Achy joints

- Insomnia

- Grinding teeth or clenching the jaw, particularly during sleep

- Upset stomach

- Racing heart, feelings of anxiety

- Breathlessness

- Dry mouth

- Headaches

- Tension in the neck and shoulders

- Sudden weight loss or gain

- Mood swings

- Decreased sexual drive

So if you need a break from the chaotic daily grind, the Urban Revitalizer Cleanse is a good way to put on the emergency brake and make time for a healing retreat. The tasty juices, energy soups and electrolyte shakes are heavy on greens, which have large amounts of chlorophyll. Chlorophyll is one of the best substances for boosting the immune system and cleansing the body's elimination systems—the digestive tract, the liver, and the blood. A few facts about chlorophyll:

∗ It has a calming effect on the body.

∗ Its molecules have magnesium at their core. Every time our heart beats, it uses magnesium, so magnesium is a critical mineral.

∗ It cleanses the blood and stimulates the production of red blood cells, which carry oxygen throughout our bodies.

∗ It has antioxidant, anti-inflammatory and wound-healing properties.

∗ It purifies the liver by helping remove old toxic material and heavy metals from the body.

∗ It helps thicken and strengthen cell walls, and (via the A, C and E vitamins) neutralizes free radicals that damage healthy cells, both of which support the immune system.

∗ It relieves both constipation and diarrhea.

Studies also show that chlorophyll may help keep carcinogens from binding to DNA in the liver and other organs. As you can see, chlorophyll is a great natural defense against the effects of stress, so get ready to green your body!

When to Do the Cleanse

If gray, pale and haggard have become part of your usual look, it's time to do the Urban Revitalizer. It's also time if caffeine has become your lifeline for staying awake and alert; if *convenience, comfort* and *to go* best describe the food you've been eating; and if life in the fast lane is getting you down or if you're feeling altogether burned out. You can do this cleanse twice each year.

What You'll See and Feel

With this cleanse, you'll have renewed energy, clarity and focus and a greater sense of serenity and a restored sense of balance in your life. As you shed the stress, you'll probably shed a few pounds as well.

REHYDRATING YOUR FACE

There's nothing like a good face spritz to rehydrate skin that gets punished by the city environment. Your face will drink it up, and the lavender and rose essential oils will chill you out.

"TRANSPORT ME TO PROVENCE" FACIAL SPRITZ

Makes about 4 ounces

1/2 cup purified water
1 drop rose essential oil
1 drop lavender essential oil
1 teaspoon raw aloe vera juice (available at local health-food stores)

Put water into 4-ounce travel-size spray bottle, then add rose and lavender essential oils and aloe juice. Put the cap back on, shake the bottle, and start spritzing!

KAREN'S TESTIMONIAL

I live life constantly on the go. Work keeps me on the road about 50% of the time, and it's rare for me to be home for a month without travel. I tend to work odd hours, sometimes in 18-hour stretches, 7 days a week. I don't have a 9-to-5 job where I can leave my work at the office and unplug at home.

Fortunately, I don't drink or smoke, but with the constant travel it's hard to get into a rhythm where I eat enough and have a balanced diet. I go through periods where all I eat are salads, nuts and protein shakes, but that's interspersed with crazy stretches on the road where I grab convenience foods that are higher in calories and lower on nutrition than I'd like. It's not uncommon that I'm too worn out to cook by the end of the day, so I go with the easy premade stuff.

Then, when I'm wiped out and need a quick boost, peanut M&M's are my vice of choice—or I'll get myself a cappuccino and a pain au chocolat. That picks me up for a bit, but then I get a dragged-out—almost drugged-out—feeling when the rush wears off. So I reach for something else with sugar or caffeine and then crash all over again. It becomes a vicious cycle.

Recently, on a particularly exhausting trip to Europe, I got food poisoning. I think the traveling, my diet and the stress on my body had worn down my resistance, and it just hit me. I bounced back from that but continued to feel achy, tired and out of sorts. I was bloated and my stomach was continually upset. My skin looked dull, and my hands and feet seemed puffy.

Having done cleanses with Adina twice before, I knew it was time to clean everything out and get my body back into balance. So I gave her a call, and she had me start the Urban Revitalizer Cleanse.

The first 24 hours were identical to what I experienced the first two times I cleansed. I got a splitting headache in the late afternoon. It peaked in the evening but was completely gone by noon the next day. I wasn't hungry that first day and had to force myself to finish the last of the juices or broths. I just felt too full—perhaps because of how well hydrated I was from drinking all the water Adina recommended.

By the second day I felt lighter. My joints were freer, not so puffy. I was still a little sluggish, but after taking a nap in the afternoon I was good to go again. Then by the third day, something really remarkable happened. I felt focused. My vision really seemed to be sharper. I'd lost at least 4 pounds, and the whites of my eyes were really clear and bright. And I started to get this very clean energy—an energized calm. I just felt balanced. For the rest of the cleanse, the energy just got better and better. I'd sleep very well and wake up ready to go.

By the end of the fourth day, I was thinking about chewing on something a bit more solid but wasn't having too hard a time. I wasn't hungry, nor was I overly full—I was simply satisfied as my appetite recalibrated to a healthier level. I experienced no cravings beyond wanting a different texture and a bit more spice.

Looking beyond the recipes, I was glad I went ahead and had a colonic. It was a real education on both a physical and spiritual level to—pardon the pun—go with the flow and clear it all out. I also had massages, dry-brushed my skin, practiced relaxation techniques, kept a journal and exercised. Together, it all increased my sense of well-being. I think you could say that as I was releasing toxins internally, the massages, walks and journaling were releasing some spiritual or psychological junk too.

By the end of the cleanse, I'd dropped 7 pounds. The bloating in my stomach was gone. I think my circulation was much better because my hands and feet weren't getting cold anymore. My skin was firmer, and it really did glow. (My friends kept asking what I was doing to make my skin so look so great!) Now that I was finally relaxed, I had no tension in my face. I looked very well rested, as if I had taken a vacation. I began to see the benefit of devoting time to really caring for myself. I had tons of energy. I felt as if my life was more balanced and calmer.

The Urban Revitalizer Cleanse gave me a lot more appreciation for the complexity of the human body. We might be able to operate on the *outside edges of balance for a long time and get by okay. But I've slowly realized that this body is the only place my soul gets to live on this Earth. It makes an incredible difference when I simply give my body the basics it needs on a consistent basis and not stress it with junk. I like ice cream and the occasional piece of cake just like everyone else—and the homemade chips from my local French café are a real treat—but it's all about moderation and keeping things in balance.*

It's so much easier to live in balance than I ever imagined. When I paid attention to putting high-quality, highly nutritious foods into my system, I got clear and energized. From there, I could see that the same thing goes for the other things you bring into your life—toxic thoughts, beliefs or people bring you down, and positive ones nurture, enrich and nourish you.

I will definitely do this again—I think of it as my personal spring cleaning!

CLEANSE AT A GLANCE*

On waking: Hot Lemon Water (see recipe on page 33)

Breakfast: Coffee-Break Green Healer Juice

Snack: Coffee-Break Green Healer Juice

Lunch: Soup of your choice

Snack: Rush-Hour Coconut Shake

Dinner: Soup of your choice

*All servings are 16 ounces.

Special Equipment

* Blender

* Juicer

* Package of cheesecloth or a muslin nut bag (nut bags are available at local health-food stores)

RECIPES

NOTE: All but one of the soup recipes in this chapter are raw soups. If chilled soups don't appeal to you, you can enjoy them at room temperature or gently heat them until just warm to preserve their enzymatic power. Young coconuts and wheatgrass shots are available at health-food stores (see page 160 for instructions on opening a young coconut).

COFFEE-BREAK GREEN HEALER JUICE

Makes 1 serving

The Green Healer gives you an enzymatic kick that energizes the body and gets the digestive juices flowing. You can add more apple for additional sweetness, or take it out completely for a low-glycemic invigorating treat!

4 or 5 celery stalks
1 cucumber
6 leaves kale or beet greens and collard greens
1 small apple (Golden Delicious)
1 tablespoon ginger
1–2 tablespoons lemon juice (or as much as you need to taste)
Optional: hint of cayenne if the weather is very cold

Chop first 5 ingredients into pieces small enough to fit into your juicer and juice them. Add the lemon juice, optional cayenne and enough water to make 16 ounces of juice. Pour into a glass and enjoy.

RUSH-HOUR COCONUT SHAKE

Makes 1 serving

This shake contains the perfect all-natural balance of water, sugar, and salt and is gentle on the stomach. If you find it too sweet, cut it with additional water. Coconut actually stimulates weight loss by increasing metabolic rate and removes harmful free radicals that promote premature aging and degenerative disease, so it's a miraculous healer! Little-known fact: coconut oil is lower in calories than all other fats. If you don't like coconut, you can enjoy a serving of Almond Milk instead (see recipe on page 93).

Milk and 4 tablespoons flesh of 1 young coconut (see directions on
   opening it below)
1/2 cup purified water

Directions: Pour coconut milk into blender. Scoop out flesh and add it to the blender. Mix together at high speed. Add more water, as needed, to make a 16-ounce serving.

OPENING A YOUNG COCONUT

To open a young coconut, use a very sharp knife to trim off as much of the outer skin off the pointy-ended top as possible. Once you reach the slightly brown, small inner shell, carefully cut into the top of the inner shell at a 45-degree angle, turning the coconut after each small slice. Once you've cut around the entire top, peel it back like the lid of a can you've opened. Pour the coconut milk into a bowl. Using a spatula, scoop out the soft flesh and add to the bowl. Discard the shell. For a video demonstration, go to www.rawguru.com.

METRO MEX AVOCADO SOUP

Makes 1 serving

This is one of my favorite soups. The zing of the spices and the crunch of the radishes wake up your taste buds, and the avocado gives it a nice creamy finish. So grab your maracas and start shaking . . . olé!

1 cup purified water
4 medium tomatoes, finely diced
1 cup cilantro, finely chopped
1 medium radish, finely diced
1 avocado, peeled, pitted and coarsely chopped
2 tablespoons fresh lime juice
1/8 teaspoon Himalayan or Celtic sea salt
1/4 teaspoon garlic, minced
1/8 teaspoon fresh ground black pepper
1 tablespoon lemon juice
1/4 teaspoon cumin
Dash of your favorite hot sauce
Optional: additional Himalayan or Celtic sea salt to taste; fresh ground
   black pepper to taste

Directions: Put first 12 ingredients into a blender. Mix until blended but not completely smooth. Add optional pepper and additional salt, as needed. Ladle into a bowl and serve.

GET-BACK-TO-GREEN SOUP

Makes 1 serving

This soup, which I created, is very popular with the clients who do the 5-day cleanse I run out of Café Gratitude in San Francisco.

They love the deep-green color and the medley of flavors that dances over your palate. If you'd like to add some variety over your 5-day cleanse, experiment with changing the flavor by adding different herbs such as dill, basil or sorrel!

1 cup purified water
1 cup cucumber, peeled and diced
2 packed cups fresh spinach leaves
¼ cup diced celery
1 cup sprouts (any sprouts will do)
½ avocado, peeled, pitted and diced
1 teaspoon chickpea or barley miso paste
Pinch of cayenne
Pinch of salt
2 tablespoons fresh lemon juice
2 tablespoons fresh cilantro, coarsely chopped
Optional: substitute 1 tablespoon chopped, fresh basil, dill or sorrel for the cilantro

Directions: Add all ingredients to a blender. Mix until blended but not completely smooth. Ladle into a bowl and serve.

CREAM-OF-COMMUTING CARROT SOUP

Makes 2 servings

This soup is orange power in a bowl! The sweetness of the carrots combined with the tang of the ginger will give you quite a liftoff. It's great if you're feeling low on energy.

1 cup carrot juice, approximately 1 pound carrots
½ cup cucumber juice, approximately 1 cucumber
½ avocado, peeled, pitted and chopped

½ cup sprouts of your choice
½ clove garlic, minced
2 teaspoons ginger, peeled and minced
½ cup purified water
1 teaspoon lime juice
Pinch of cayenne pepper and Himalayan or Celtic sea salt

Directions: Place all ingredients in a blender and process until smooth and creamy.

BRIDGE-AND-TUNNEL GREEN SOUP

Makes 1 serving

This soup is surprisingly satisfying, chock-full of energy and simply delicious.

1 cup purified water
1 cup spinach, washed and cut into bite-sized pieces
½ cup sprouts
1 teaspoon jalapeño, deseeded and minced
1 tablespoon lemon juice
4 raw macadamia nuts
½ large avocado, peeled and pitted
⅛ teaspoon Himalayan or Celtic sea salt

Directions: Put all ingredients into a blender and process until smooth. Ladle into a bowl and serve.

PDA PEPPER SOUP

Makes 1 serving

This soup reminds me of my summers living in northern California on the Eel River. The contrasts between the nutty, spicy arugula, the sweet red pepper and the creamy avocado are a real hit with clients and friends.

1 cup purified water
1 cup red pepper, cut into large dice
1/2 cup peeled cucumber, cut into large dice
1 tablespoon minced yellow onion
1/2 large avocado, pitted and peeled
1 tablespoon basil, chopped
1 teaspoon Bragg Liquid Aminos
Pinch of red pepper flakes or turmeric

Directions: Put all ingredients into a blender and pulse until well mixed, but still chunky. Ladle into a bowl and serve.

ROCK-THE-CASBAH SOUP

Makes 1 serving

This creamy almond soup is high in protein and packed with energy. The flavors come to life with the wine vinegar and chili flakes!

1 1/2 cups spinach or arugula, or a combination
1/2 cup almond milk
1/2 cup celery, chopped
1/2 cup sunflower or mung bean sprouts (or both—we love sprouts!)

Pinch of red chili flakes
1 tablespoon minced green onions
1 cup water
1 teaspoon umeboshi vinegar

Directions: Blend all ingredients together in a blender until smooth. Pour into a bowl and serve.

Cleanse-Boosting Activities

Play in the Dirt

Relax the pace of your urban lifestyle by getting back in touch with the Earth—literally! Volunteer at a community garden, find an organic farm outside the city where you can pick vegetables or fruit, or plant a mini herb garden on your kitchen windowsill or balcony. Having your hands and feet in the soil will help you get more . . . grounded.

You can also spend an hour or an afternoon in a park, sitting against a tree or walking barefoot in the grass. Tour a botanical garden or arboretum. In the evening, sit on a deck, a fire escape, or a roof and look at the moon and the stars. If you're able to get out of town, head to the beach, mountains, forest or desert—anywhere where you'll be surrounded by nature.

Wherever you choose to go, take it all in using different senses. Appreciate the beauty you see around you. Run your hands through the grass, plants or sand. Feel the breeze in your face. Listen to the wind or birds. Breathe in the serenity around you as you exhale any stress or burdens you've been carrying around.

Devoting this time to consciously disconnecting from city stimuli and reconnecting with the rhythms of nature will have a calming effect on your body and your state of mind.

Unplug from Stressful, Toxic Energy

Be selective about the images and information you put in your mind (and spirit) during the cleanse. Put down the paper, shut off the TV, and stop surfing the Internet—explore what it feels like not to be influenced by media and the electronic world. If there are relationships in your life that increase stress, disconnect from them during the cleanse as well—and think about whether they're helping or hurting your well-being in the longer term.

Feel the Splendor in the Grass

A combination of guided meditation and deep breathing is an excellent way to alleviate stress—you lower your heart rate, drop your blood pressure, increase the circulation of oxygen through your body and clear your mind. It will help you unwind before bedtime, but you can also do it anytime during the day. Start by lying comfortably on the floor. (Lying on a yoga mat or rug might make it more comfortable for you—have a blanket nearby, in case you get cold.) Maintain the natural curvature of your spine by keeping your cervical and lumbar vertebrae slightly off the floor (you should have enough room to slip your fingers between the floor and your lower back and the floor and your neck). If your lower back is uncomfortable, place a rolled-up towel under your knees. Check in with yourself and notice where you feel tension or stress in your body. Consciously try to relax those muscles.

Now, close your eyes and imagine that the floor beneath you is a green field covered with wildflowers. Hear the sounds of nature around you. Feel the gentle breeze playing in the grass and caressing your body. Relax into the calmness of that field. Once you're there, place a hand on your abdomen and take a deep, gentle breath through your nose, filling your belly and then your chest. Exhale through your nose, emptying your chest and belly. Let go of all the air you can without straining yourself. As you repeat these deep, soothing breaths, imagine the stress, burdens or feelings you've been carrying around peeling off your body and seeping into the earth below you. Repeat until you feel that your body has completely relaxed.

Strike a Pose

For 5,000 years, yoga has been used to relax the body and mind. I recommend doing the easy, stress-reducing yoga posture, or asana, included below at a time that works for you during the day. It's just as good as a bedtime story to help you get to sleep at night!

SAVASANA

Savasana is the ideal position for the Splendor in the Grass guided meditation and breathing exercise mentioned on page 166. Done correctly, it can release muscular, nervous, mental and emotional tensions almost immediately, allowing your body to recharge its battery. The posture is a natural tranquilizer that can help you overcome insomnia and foster a restful sleep.

Instructions

1 Lie flat on your back, maintaining the natural curvature of the spine (see the Splendor in the Grass exercise).

2 Stretch your legs out, knees slightly flexed and legs spread comfortably apart. If you feel any strain on your lower back, put a rolled-up towel under your knees.

3 Extend the arms, palms up, and rest them on the floor away from the sides of your body.

4 Relax your jaw, allowing your mouth to fall open slightly and letting your teeth part a bit.

5 Close your eyes and breathe naturally through the nose, making no attempt to regulate your breathing.

6 Lie quietly, letting your muscles relax completely.

7 Let go of any stress or concerns burdening your mind.

8 If you find that parts of your body are still tense, make a conscious effort to release the muscles.

9 Focus solely on your breath until you lose awareness of your physical body.

10 When you're done, stretch your limbs and move slowly to a seated position before standing up.

THE WINTER WAKE-UP CLEANSE (5 TO 7 DAYS)

Winter and the holiday season can be a period of reflection and celebration. We spend time with people we love, we look back on the past, and we set our intentions for the future. On the flip side, this time of year can leave us feeling lethargic if we indulge in heavy foods, meat, desserts and alcohol at gatherings and parties. We're often less active, staying inside to avoid the cold weather. It's no surprise that this combination depletes our energy and leaves us susceptible to illness (and it can make our waistbands a bit snug, too).

Historically, Eastern medicine prescribed cleanses only during the spring, summer or fall. In ancient times, humans were much more in tune with the cycles of nature: When winter came, the shorter days curbed our activity and we became more sedentary, and to keep warm and survive we had to put on a few pounds. It was the human version of hibernating.

But thousands of years later, we live in a very different world where modern conveniences have diminished the impact of the seasons on our lives. I firmly believe we need to reconnect with nature and resync our internal clocks with the seasons. However, these days very few of us need to worry about gaining weight to stay alive in the wintertime, and the amount of refined foods and sugars that we consume—particularly around the holidays—is toxic to our bodies. So we really don't have to wait for warmer months to do a cleanse in today's world. We might just need to put on a hat, socks and an extra sweater as we detox!

To help heat this cleanse up for the winter months, I've added ginger and cayenne to the recipes to keep you warm and cleanse your blood. I've also included a mineral broth to heat the body and bones on chilly winter evenings.

The green juices in this cleanse are rich in chlorophyll and low in natural sugars. As mentioned in the chapter about the Urban Revitalizer Cleanse, chlorophyll has some wide-ranging health benefits: It stops the growth of fungus, yeast, and bad bacteria in the intestinal tract; removes drug deposits; and detoxifies the liver, just to name a few (see page 154). Green juices also emulsify cholesterol and fat in the body.

If you find yourself feeling stuck or unwell early in the year, the Winter Wake-Up is the perfect antidote to the effects of a post-holiday food coma. But, be forewarned: it's not one I recommend starting with if you've never detoxed before. The Winter Wake-Up is predominantly a juice cleanse, so it's fairly intense. Just how intense will depend on your regular diet and current digestive health. It's normal to experience a host of healing reactions, outlined in the "Get Ready . . . Get Set . . ." chapter (see page 7). After a few days, you'll feel much better and should get relief from the cravings for unhealthy foods, sugar, caffeine, tobacco and more. As you rebound, you'll feel a steady increase in your energy and may even experience a sense of euphoria that's typical during a serious cleanse.

If you *are* physically and mentally prepared for a rigorous cleanse, the Winter Wake-Up will leave you energized and rejuvenated at every level. It's a perfect way to clean your slate and set your intentions for a healthier, happier year ahead.

When to Do the Cleanse

If you're experiencing post-holiday toxic shock and weight gain from overeating, too much drinking, and underexercising, it's time to do the Winter Wake-Up Cleanse. Do the cleanse if you want to break an addiction to sugar, if you feel as if your life force has gone underground to hibernate, if you've been catching every cold or flu bug that crosses your path, or if you're just itching for an early inner spring!

It's called the Winter Wake-Up, but you can do it twice in a year.

What You'll See and Feel

This cleanse will fuel new levels of energy, clarity and lightness into your life. You'll feel rejuvenated on every level—in fact, many of my clients report feeling euphoric. In addition, the boost in hydration and nutrients will ease the dry skin and lips so common in wintertime and get you glowing again.

BUDDY UP!

The Winter Wake-Up is a serious cleanse and there's quite a bit of juicing involved, so I strongly recommend doing this with a friend. You can check in with each other to provide support during the detox phase, and you can take turns being the chef. Maybe one of you rises with the sun and the other is at his or her best after the sun sets—let the early bird juice in the morning and have the night owl take the evening shift. Maybe you'll decide to trade off kitchen duty every other day. Or perhaps you'll be really ambitious and have a juice-off! Do whatever works for you. Just know it can make a big difference to share the experience and the work.

ELIZA'S TESTIMONIAL

*Coming off the winter holidays in 2005 was a real eye-opener for me.
For 6 straight weeks, it was one big party—lots of great and seriously
decadent food, and plenty of spirits to toast the holidays and ring in the
New Year. I had my usual good fun. But this time around, I felt as if
I had the world's worst, unending hangover once the holidays had
passed.*

*I didn't feel well. I was really cranky. Mentally, it was as if I were
walking through quicksand. I felt totally spent, even if I'd just slept for
8 hours. And I had hit the "big 4-0" weighing 25 pounds more than I
did 5 years earlier. In the cold winter light, it was not a pretty picture.
This was not me—or at least it wasn't the me I remembered or wanted
to be. I wanted to feel well and content and get my energy back.*

*I went to an Ayurvedic practitioner who recommended that I sign
up to do one of Adina's cleanses. I'd never done one before, so I wasn't
100% sure it was the route to go, but I was desperate to do something
to get the ball rolling. I made the mistake of ignoring advice and
jumped right into a pretty aggressive cleanse, so the first couple of days
were rough. I had headaches, I was hungry and I woke up with pain-
ful cramps in the middle of the first night as the juices and broth began
to seriously flush out my system.*

*But I stuck with it, and by the end of the second day I started to feel
different. I wasn't craving my usual food, and I actually felt full.
I started sleeping really soundly, and my energy began to pick up. I was
thinking more clearly. By day 3, I could even see a difference in my
appearance—my eyes looked brighter and my skin looked pinker and
healthier.*

*But the biggest surprise wasn't what I experienced physically, which
was awesome; it was what I experienced in my head and heart. Without the crutch of comfort foods, I had to deal with a lot of buried emotions that started to surface. I started to get back in touch with myself.
I felt calmer and more centered and really awake.*

I had no idea that it would be such a transformative experience: I'm still eating differently a year later and loving it. The Winter Wake-Up is amazing!

CLEANSE AT A GLANCE*

On Waking: Hot Lemon Water (see recipe on page 33)

Breakfast: Green juice of your choice

Snack: Green juice of your choice and a wheatgrass shot

Lunch: Thaw-Me-Out Yam Broth or Taste of Thai Soup

Snack: Green juice of your choice

Dinner: Thaw-Me-Out Yam Broth or Taste of Thai Soup

Snack: Green juice of your choice

*If you find you need to chew on something, you can snack on your choice of a small handful of almonds (which have been soaked in water overnight), celery sticks or cucumber slices a few times a day. But be sure to chew them very well to aid in digestion!

Special Equipment

* Juicer
* High-Speed Blender

RECIPES

The green juices in this chapter are pure energy in a glass. Unlike what you get with a cup of coffee, the kick you get with the juices is even, sustained, and balanced—and there's no caffeine crash. If you're new to green juices, the flavor may take some time to grow on you. It's always a good idea to dilute the juice with some water and squeeze in a bit more lemon juice, to taste.

To get the most out of these concoctions, buy your produce from a local farmers' market. Organic greens straight from the field have the most nutrients, and they're free of pesticides and chemical fertilizers. This is particularly important because you don't peel all fruits and vegetables before juicing. Most of the nutrients are packed in the skin!

> NOTE: Burdock root, kombu and wheatgrass are available at health-food stores. Dandelion greens are available at many grocery stores and specialty markets.

WINTER NECTAR

Makes 1 serving

½ head celery (4–5 stalks)
1 beet
5 kale leaves (any type)
1–2 teaspoons fresh ginger
1 cucumber
Fresh lemon juice to taste

Directions: Chop first 5 ingredients into pieces small enough to fit into the feed tube of your juicer. Juice each of the ingredients, starting with the beet and ending with the cucumber, to ensure that you get every drop of juice from the kale and ginger. Pour into a glass, add water as needed to make 16 ounces, and serve with a wedge or two of lemon.

SPRUCE JUICE

Makes 1 serving

1 cucumber
2 dandelion green leaves
5 collard green leaves
8 celery stalks
1 pear, cored
Fresh lemon juice to taste

Directions: Chop first 5 ingredients into pieces small enough to fit into the feed tube of your juicer. Juice each of the ingredients, starting with the cucumber and ending with the celery and pear, to ensure that you get every drop of juice from the dandelion leaves and collard greens. Pour into a glass, add water as needed to make 16 ounces, and serve with a wedge or two of lemon.

GREEN MACHINE

Makes one 16-ounce serving

1 head celery (8–10 stalks)
2 cups spinach leaves
1 teaspoon fresh ginger
1 green apple, cored

Directions: Chop ingredients into pieces small enough to fit into the feed tube of your juicer. Juice each of the ingredients, starting with the celery and ending with the apple, to ensure that you get every drop of juice from the spinach and ginger. Pour into a glass, add water as needed to make 16 ounces, and serve.

THE GREAT VEGGIE MATE

Makes 1 serving

I love using sunflower sprouts in this recipe, but you can also use clover, alfalfa, or any other young, fresh sprout you're able to find.

4 carrots
1 cup sprouts
5 chard leaves
2 heads romaine lettuce
1 cucumber
1 lime, peel removed
1 pinch of Himalayan or Celtic sea salt
1 pinch of cayenne pepper (very hot—a little goes a long way)

Directions: Chop the first 6 ingredients into pieces small enough to fit into the feed tube of your juicer. Juice each of the ingredients, starting with the carrots and ending with the cucumber, to ensure that you get every drop of juice from the sprouts and chard. Stir in the lime juice, salt and cayenne. Pour into a glass, add water as needed to make 16 ounces, and serve.

THE SHAMROCK

Makes 1 serving

1 cucumber
5 celery stalks
2 kale leaves
2 chard leaves
1 small lemon, peeled
2 or 3 parsley sprigs
1 small fennel bulb

Directions: Chop all ingredients into pieces small enough to fit into the feed tube of your juicer. Juice each of the ingredients, starting with the cucumber and celery and ending with the fruit and fennel, to ensure that you get every drop of juice from the kale, chard and parsley. Pour into a glass, add water as needed to make 16 ounces, and serve.

THAW-ME-OUT YAM BROTH

Makes 4 servings

Broth is a wonder food. It's a great-tasting way to get loads of essential minerals and vitamins in a way that's easy to digest. This broth can be made in advance; it will last up to 3 days in the refrigerator. The optional medicinal herbs pack a powerful cleansing punch.

2 cups celery, chopped (3 or 4 stalks)
2 cups yellow onions, chopped (about 2 medium onions)
2 cups leeks, chopped (about 1 large leek or 2 medium leeks)
*1 cup fresh burdock root, chopped (about a 6- to 8-inch piece of
   burdock root)*
One 4-inch piece kombu, chopped
4 tablespoons fresh ginger, chopped
2 cups carrots, chopped (about 3 medium carrots)
10 cloves garlic, separated, but not peeled
12 sprigs parsley
3 medium yams, washed and cut in half
Himalayan or Celtic sea salt to taste
Cayenne pepper to taste
*Optional: 1 teaspoon fresh gingerroot, peeled and minced; 1 table-
   spoon red clover blossom; 1 tablespoon sage; or 1 tablespoon
   yellow dock root*

Directions: In a 5-quart stockpot, combine the celery, onions, leeks, burdock root, kombu, ginger, carrots, garlic cloves, parsley and yams, leaving the yams on top. Add cold water up to 1 inch from the top of the pot. Bring to a boil, then reduce the heat. Simmer the broth on the stove top for 1½ hours. Turn heat off and let broth cool for at least 30 minutes. When broth is cool, pull out the yams and set them aside. Strain the broth through a colander into a bowl. Discard the remaining vegetables. In small batches, purée the liquid broth and pieces of yam in a blender until you get a light soup consistency. Add salt and cayenne to taste. (Be careful—a little goes a long way!) Add the optional teaspoon of minced fresh ginger, red clover blossoms, sage or yellow dock root if you'd like more heat and flavor. Reheat portions until warm and serve.

TASTE OF THAI SOUP

Makes 4 servings

This soup puts a twist on traditional Thai tom yum gung soup. Ingredients such as coriander, lemongrass and galangal root are quite medicinal. In fact, a recent joint study by Thailand's Kasetsart University and Japan's Kyoto and Kinki Universities has found that the ingredients in tom yum gung soup are 100 times more effective in inhibiting cancerous tumor growth than other foods. In addition, the spiciness of the dish is sure to keep your taste buds satisfied and your body warm in the wintertime.

3 stalks lemongrass
10 cups purified water
2 cups celery, chopped
1 cup fresh tomatoes, chopped
2 medium onions, cut in half
5 tablespoons fresh ginger, minced

10 cloves garlic, peeled
1 cup cilantro, destemmed
1 small butternut or kabocha squash
2 medium carrots, thinly sliced
1¼ inches fresh or frozen galangal root, cut into five ¼-inch slices
Fresh lime juice to taste
Red chili paste to taste (very hot—use sparingly)
Garnish: 3 scallion tops, thinly sliced

Directions: Take ⅔ off the top of each lemongrass stalk and discard. Peel away outer layers of the remaining pieces, cut each one into 3 pieces, and "bruise" with the back of a cleaver. In a 5-quart stockpot, combine the lemongrass and next 10 ingredients. Bring to a boil, then reduce the heat and simmer for 90 minutes. Turn heat off and let broth cool for at least 30 minutes. When cooled, take out the pieces of squash and set them aside. Strain the broth through a colander into a large bowl. Discard the rest of the vegetables. In small batches, mix a combination of the liquid broth and pieces of the squash in a blender until you get a light broth consistency. Add lime juice and chili paste to taste. Ladle into a bowl, garnish with scallions, and enjoy!

Cleanse-Boosting Activities

Get to the Point

If winter has left you feeling stuck or low on energy, a Shiatsu massage—also called acupressure—is a great way to get your life force flowing again. It's a Japanese form of physical therapy based on the Chinese medical theory that disease and pain are caused by blocked qi (energy) along energy meridians in the body. Shiatsu practitioners combine massage, gentle stretching and pressure to the meridian points to open blocked lines of energy and restore and maintain balance in the body. It's the most reviving form of massage I've ever experienced!

Take the Plunge

If you've been hibernating for the winter, a hot–cold plunge—or hydrotherapy—is one of the best ways to invigorate yourself. In hydrotherapy, you alternate between submerging yourself in a pool of hot water and submerging in a pool of cold water. It's been a common practice for hundreds of years in cultures around the world because of its recuperative, healing effects. The hot and cold stimuli carry the impulses felt at the skin deeper into the body, where they stimulate the immune system, block the production of stress-producing hormones, improve circulation and digestion, and lessen sensitivity to pain. Call local spas and gyms to see who might offer hydrotherapy in your area.

Sow Seeds for Spring

It's wintertime, so find ways to create warmth in your home. If you have a fireplace, use it. Build a roaring fire and sit in front of it in the evening, sipping tea or warm soup. No fireplace? No problem. Light an assortment of candles—they generate more heat than you might imagine and create an inviting radiance in the room. If you use your favorite naturally scented candles, you'll add soothing aromatherapy to the warm, wonderful glow!

While you're basking in the candlelight or firelight, think of some area of your life or a relationship where you'd like a fresh start. What would it look like if you were starting from a clean slate? How would that feel? What would be different? What are two or three tangible things you could do to get there? Sow these seeds of intention now so you can breathe new life into the situation when the winter thaws.

THE GREEN BUZZ CLEANSE (5 TO 7 DAYS)

Each of the preceding cleanses are stepping-stones leading to the Green Buzz, because when it comes to cleanses, it's the closest program to fasting in this book. This super-healing cleanse is so effective because the life-giving nutrients are delivered in raw, liquid form—flushing your system far more rapidly than the other cleanses in this book.

The high levels of chlorophyll from the green vegetables and algae in the Green Buzz juice recipes are liquid sunshine for the body: They alkalize the body; boost the immune system; act as an anti-inflammatory; remove carcinogens and drug deposits; counteract the effects of radiation; help stop the growth of bacteria, yeast and fungus; increase alertness; and emulsify cholesterol and fat. Greens are also chock-full of the enzymes, vitamins, minerals and antioxidants our body needs to protect and heal itself.

And as the Green Buzz clears waste and the acid it produces from your body, your muscles relax and cellular enzymes function better. Dead cells are purged from the body, and the blood, organs and tissues are rejuvenated. Bloat melts from your body and face. Fog clears from your brain and spirit. Dark circles under your eyes are erased, luster returns to your skin, and the signs of aging appear to reverse. Stress and tension ease as the natural antidepressant effects of the chlorophyll kick in.

Because the detox (or healing) reactions during this cleanse can be stronger than what you'd experience with other cleanses, the Green Buzz requires a total commitment to healing and rejuvenating yourself. That's particularly true if you've long had a poor diet or partake in other vices (tobacco, caffeine, alcohol, etc.). If you've been eating a "clean" whole-foods diet, you may not experience any of these symptoms. In any case, reread the healing reactions outlined on page 7 so that you're prepared.

For most clients, I recommend building up to the Green Buzz by trying the "Some Like It Raw," Laughing Buddha or Three-Day Face-Lift cleanses first. Doing this cleanse requires willpower and commitment, so I recommend finding a friend to do the cleanse with you: You can give each other moral support during the detox phase, talk about what you're experiencing and maybe even share the work of juicing! I also recommend consulting your physician, in advance, to talk about this cleanse in light of medications you might be taking or preexisting conditions you might have.

If you're ready for the Green Buzz, don't compromise here— follow the cleanse as prescribed! It'll take some work, but the extent of the healing you'll experience is worth it. Once you get through the detox phase, you'll notice that you have more energy, think more clearly, sleep more soundly, and wake up alert and ready to start the day. You'll also be happy with the changes in your appearance—clearer eyes, fewer lines on your face, and luminous skin from head to toe. You'll probably notice that you've shed some pounds as well.

When it comes to your palate and the way you think about what you eat, the Green Buzz will pave the way to a fresh, healthier relationship with food.

When to Do the Cleanse

When you want to restore a healthy color, glow and tone to your skin, you're ready for the Green Buzz. You'll benefit from it when you want to achieve a higher level of energy, clarity and vitality; when you're battling health issues and want to try a natural alternative or supplement for healing the body; when you want to start over and experience a total metamorphosis! This all-juice cleanse is appropriate to do once or twice a year.

NOTE: Because it's an all-juice cleanse that's cooling to the body, I recommend doing the Green Buzz during the warmer months of the year.

What You'll See and Feel

The Green Buzz brings a marked boost in energy and clarity and a lightness to the body, mind and spirit. Bloat should melt away and flexibility can increase dramatically. Many people feel a sense of ease and deeper awareness of and compassion for others and themselves. The cleanse can also create a strong sense of empowerment and accomplishment.

ELIZABETH'S TESTIMONIAL

In 1995, my breast cancer was diagnosed; I was 35 years old. Up to that point, I had a hectic lifestyle, working two jobs. I was a chef in a high-end San Francisco restaurant and a physical therapist in a rehab hospital caring for patients with brain and spinal cord injuries. I thought I'd led a pretty healthy life—I was in great shape from mountain biking and lifting patients 4 to 6 hours a day, and

I'd been eating lots of fresh vegetables and fish. But in hindsight, I can also see that I consumed a lot of processed sugars, wine and caffeine and I rarely sat down to enjoy a meal. My pace of life and diet had been quietly undermining my health.

After dealing with the toxicity of surgical anesthesia and 6 months of chemotherapy, I was completely exhausted. My skin was gray, I had a metallic taste in my mouth, and I was bloated and constipated. To supplement the chemotherapy, I sought out Eastern medical practices such as acupuncture and Reiki and also did colonics. My colon hydrotherapist suggested I do a wheatgrass-and-green-juice cleanse to help flush the toxic chemicals and recalibrate my body.

So I signed up for a 7-day cleanse at a retreat center. The second and third day weren't easy—I was fatigued, bored, mentally foggy, craving food and riding an emotional roller coaster. But after surviving chemo, I knew I could get through this. I added Epsom salts baths to help calm my body before bed and draw toxins from my skin, and I carried on.

By day 4, I felt a shift—I was no longer hungry and I'd started shedding some pounds. By the end of the week, the results were miraculous: I'd completely lost the bloat (my pants were loose!), the metallic taste in my mouth was gone and my skin looked vibrant. I felt as if the vibration had shifted in every cell of my body—I had tons of energy and amazing mental clarity. I've done cleanses twice a year since then to keep my body on track. More than 12 years later, I'm still cancer-free.

That cleanse changed my life. I left the restaurant and rehab facility to focus my work on creating cleansing foods and opening my own catering business. Along the way, I met Adina. On the basis of our work and personal experiences, we knew an all-juice fast wasn't for everyone. So we decided to combine our knowledge to create a cleanse that was more warming and filling. The end result was a predecessor of her Winter Wake-Up.

I encourage anyone thinking about cleansing to consider it a vacation for their digestive tract. Expect and look forward to the profound *shift you're going to experience rather than focusing on the fact that you won't be eat like you usually do—it's so much easier that way. It's a gift you give to your body, and your body will thank you!*

CLEANSE AT A GLANCE

You can drink a juice every 3 hours, but you might find you don't need that much in a day. If the juice-only regimen becomes too much for you, you can eat some peeled cucumber or a few almonds that have been soaked in water overnight, but chew them very thoroughly.

On waking: Hot Lemon Water (see recipe on page 33)

Every 3 hours: Juice of your choice

Throughout the day: Water, herbal teas and wheatgrass

Special Equipment

* Blender
* Juicer
* Tongue scraper

RECIPES

While you are doing the Green Buzz, it's particularly important to buy organic produce that's free of pesticides and chemical fertilizers. As long as you buy organic produce, you don't have to worry about peeling your vegetables before juicing.

If you're new to green juices, the flavor may take some time to grow on you. I've included fruit in several of the recipes to take some of the bite out of the greens. You can also dilute the juice with some additional water and squeeze in a bit more lemon or lime juice, to taste. You can add 1 teaspoon blue-green algae to your juice to pump up the chlorophyll and add protein.

NOTE: Blue-green algae, spirulina and wheatgrass are available at local health-food stores. Dandelion greens are available at many grocery stores and specialty markets.

THE GRASSHOPPER

Makes 1 serving

1 cucumber
½ head celery (4–5 stalks)
5 or 6 kale leaves
1 small beet
1 teaspoon fresh lime juice

Directions: Chop the first 4 ingredients into pieces small enough to fit into the feed tube of your juicer. Juice each of the ingredients, starting with the cucumber and ending with the beet, to ensure you get every drop of juice from the kale. Pour into a glass, and add lime juice and enough water to bring the juice up to 16 ounces. Stir and enjoy.

COOL JUICE

Makes 1 serving

1 cucumber
One 1-inch piece fresh ginger, peeled
7 parsley sprigs
1 small romaine lettuce head
5 kale leaves
3 large carrots
2 teaspoons fresh lemon juice

Directions: Chop the first 6 ingredients into pieces small enough to fit into the feed tube of your juicer. Juice each of the ingredients, starting with the cucumber and ending with the carrots, to ensure that you get every drop of juice from the ginger, parsley and lettuce. Pour into a glass and add lemon juice and enough water to bring the juice up to 16 ounces. Stir and enjoy.

FARMER BROWN'S ELIXIR

Makes 1 serving

1 cucumber
1 head celery (8–10 stalks)
5 collard greens or dandelion green leaves
2 large tomatoes
1 pinch of cayenne pepper

Directions: Chop the first 4 ingredients into pieces small enough to fit into the feed tube of your juicer. Juice each of the ingredients, starting with the cucumber and ending with the tomato, to ensure that you get every drop of juice from the collard greens or dandelion. Pour into a glass and add enough water to bring the juice up to 16 ounces. Stir and enjoy.

PIRATE'S POTION

Makes 1 serving

1 head celery (8–10 stalks)
2 cups fresh spinach
1 tomato
One 2-inch piece of fresh ginger, peeled
1 large cucumber

1 cup sprouts
½ cup parsley
2 teaspoons fresh lime juice

Directions: Chop the first 5 ingredients into pieces small enough to fit into the feed tube of your juicer. Juice each of the ingredients, starting with the celery and ending with the cucumber, to ensure that you get every drop of juice from the spinach, ginger, sprouts and parsley. Pour into a glass, stir in lime juice, and add enough water—as needed—to bring the juice up to 16 ounces. Stir and enjoy.

RAINBOW BLEND

Makes 1 serving

1 cucumber
4 large carrots
5 chard leaves
1 head celery (8–10 stalks)
1 beet
1 teaspoon fresh lemon juice
Pinch of cayenne pepper (be careful to make it a small pinch!)

Directions: Chop the first 5 ingredients into pieces small enough to fit into the feed tube of your juicer. Juice each of the ingredients, starting with the cucumber and ending with the beet, to ensure that you get every drop of juice from the chard. Pour into a glass and add lemon juice and cayenne. Add enough water—as needed—to bring the juice up to 16 ounces. Stir and enjoy.

SOUTH OF THE BORDER

Makes 1 serving

1 cucumber
1 tomato
1 red pepper, seeded
5 cilantro sprigs
1 large carrot
1 head celery (8–10 stalks)
1 teaspoon fresh lime juice
Pinch of Himalayan or Celtic sea salt

Directions: Chop the first 6 ingredients into pieces small enough to fit into the feed tube of your juicer. Juice each of the ingredients, starting with the cucumber and ending with the celery, to ensure that you get every drop of juice from the cilantro. Pour into a glass and add lime juice and salt. Add enough water—as needed—to bring the juice up to 16 ounces. Stir and enjoy.

APPLE TURNOVER

Makes 1 serving

½ head celery (4–5 stalks)
1 apple, cored
5 kale leaves
2 cucumbers
2 teaspoons fresh lemon juice

Directions: Chop the first 4 ingredients into pieces small enough to fit into the feed tube of your juicer. Juice each of the ingredients, starting with the celery and ending with the cucumber, to ensure that you get every drop of juice from the kale. Pour into a glass and add the lemon juice. Add enough water—as needed—to bring the juice up to 16 ounces. Stir and enjoy.

WATERMELON GREENS

Makes 1 serving

2 cups watermelon flesh, cubed
5 chard leaves
1 cucumber

Directions: Chop the ingredients into pieces small enough to fit into the feed tube of your juicer. Juice each of the ingredients, starting with the watermelon and ending with the cucumber, to ensure that you get every drop of juice from the chard. Pour into a glass and enjoy.

THE RABBIT

Makes 1 serving

1 head romaine lettuce
1 cup sprouts
½ cup arugula
5 cilantro sprigs
5 kale leaves
6 large carrots
1 teaspoon fresh lime juice

Directions: Chop the first 6 ingredients into pieces small enough to fit into the feed tube of your juicer. Juice each of the ingredients, starting and ending with the carrots, to ensure that you get every drop of juice from the sprouts, arugula, cilantro and kale. Pour into a glass and add lime juice. Add enough water—as needed—to bring the juice up to 16 ounces. Stir and enjoy.

APPLE PROTEIN SUPER GREEN JUICE

Makes 1 serving

2 apples, cored
1 cucumber
⅛ teaspoon or 1 capsule green powder
1 teaspoon fresh lemon juice

Directions: Chop the apple and cucumber into pieces small enough to fit into the feed tube of your juicer. Juice them. Pour into a glass and add green powder and lemon juice. Add enough water—as needed—to bring the juice up to 16 ounces. Stir and enjoy.

Cleanse-Boosting Activities

Feed Your Sense of Smell

During the Green Buzz, treat yourself with aromatherapy and essential oils. You can add them to body lotion or bathwater, or refresh an entire room by adding a few drops of oil to an aromatherapy diffuser. Certain smells soothe and calm; others stimulate and awaken the brain and body. If you're feeling adventurous, combine a few oils to make your own scent: geranium rose and lavender are a great relaxing combination; ylang-ylang and cinnamon are arousing together; and orange and bergamot pair up for a peppy, energizing scent.

Stick Out Your Tongue and Say "Aaah"

When your body goes through a serious cleanse, you'll probably notice a white coating on your tongue. This is a normal sign that you're detoxing. To freshen your breath and get rid of the film, use a tongue scraper every morning before you brush your teeth. They're inexpensive and easy to use, and you can find them at local health-food stores.

Search Your Sole

When you do the Green Buzz Cleanse it is a great time to get a reflexology foot massage. The pressure points on the feet correspond to all of the glands, organs and systems in your body. Reflexology stimulates your energy, releases stress, relaxes stressed organs and facilitates the purification process. Check with your local massage therapist, a Chinese medicine practitioner or a holistic healing center for a referral to a good reflexologist.

Get "Hands-Off" Healing

As you're flushing toxins from your body, take the opportunity to clear out blocked energy and emotions through a Reiki treatment. The meaning of *Reiki* (pronounced "ray-key") is "universal life force." Reiki is an ancient art of healing that shares its roots with acupuncture and Shiatsu massage. In Reiki, a practitioner places his or her hands above parts of the body, transmitting life energy into the client's body to treat the whole person, including body, mind and spirit. The belief is that the energy heals the spirit, which then heals the body. If you've never done energy work done before, it's amazing. When I've had a Reiki session, it's felt like heat or tingling radiating from the areas in the greatest need of healing, followed by a soothing sense of peace and well-being. It's like the slate's been cleaned of old baggage, aches and pains, and stress. And it can be especially helpful in alleviating the detox symptoms you might experience during the first couple of days of the Green Buzz.

"THERE'S NO PLACE LIKE HOME" CLEANSE

A book about cleansing the body without a chapter about the toxins in our homes would be an incomplete picture, because we inhale or absorb the chemicals that we use on our skin, hair, teeth, clothes, kitchens, bathrooms, floors and furniture. We wouldn't dream of drinking a household cleaner, but those chemicals can leach into our bodies through the skin or lungs. Do we really know what's in the products we use every day?

According to the World Resources Institute, 17,000 chemicals appear in common household products. Only 30% of them have been adequately tested for their negative effects on our health and nothing is known about the combined effects of these chemicals when mixed within our bodies. And an article in *U.S. News & World Report* estimates that we're exposed to 200 chemicals a day through personal care products alone—a fact that's even more unsettling when you consider that U.S. law allows companies to put virtually any ingredient into these products with no required premarket safety testing.

The fact is, a lifetime of habit combined with a general lack of knowledge has made it easy for us to stock our cabinets with harmful chemicals that hide behind the promises of a clean home and a beautiful body. Slowly, the toxins in these products can affect the way we look and feel. Bottom line: what's around us is also within us.

HIDDEN HAZARDS

The harmful chemicals in products we use are too numerous to list—and there's been little research done on the cumulative effect of exposure to all these chemicals—but here's a snapshot of a few of the bad eggs:

- Alkylphenoxypolyethoxy ethanols, found in many laundry detergents, have been linked with breast cancer.

- Sodium hypochlorate, found in household bleach and cleaners, combines with organic compounds in the environment and has been tied to reproductive, endocrine and immune disorders.

- Formaldehyde, phenol and naphthalene, used in many air fresheners, have been connected to cancer, birth defects, and neurological damage.

- Sodium lauryl phosphates, the foaming agent found in many toothpastes, is also used commercially to degrease engines and has been tied to mouth ulcers and canker sores. Triclosan, an antimicrobial agent added to many toothpastes, has been linked to skin irritation, allergies, resistance to antibiotics and dioxin contamination.

- Dioxins, a byproduct of the process of bleaching tampons, have been linked to cancer and reproductive problems. Organic tampons are a safer bet.

In this cleanse, we clue in to what's in the products we use day in and day out, figure out what we can get rid of, and replace them with biologically friendly concoctions that get the job done without negatively affecting our bodies or the Earth. If you've come this far and made a commitment to doing a dietary cleanse, why not take it one step further and purge the skull and crossbones from your kitchen and bathroom cabinets?

When to Do the Cleanse

If you want your home environment to be as clean as your post-dietary-cleanse body, this cleanse is for you. It's time to do this cleanse if you're suffering chronic mystery allergies or ailments; if you're having reactions such as headaches, congestion, dizziness or fatigue after using specific products and it's starting to feel suspect to you; and if you want to be a more conscious consumer.

What You'll See and Feel

When you do this cleanse, you'll experience a sense of lightness, relief and empowerment that rivals any spring cleaning you've done in the past. You'll have a heightened sense of smell, a newfound peace and trust in knowing your home is safer and healthier, and a stronger connection to the Earth. With the decrease of toxins in your home environment, you may also notice that unexplained malaise, headaches, sore throats, skin conditions, respiratory issues, immune problems and/or fatigue fade away.

BETHANY'S TESTIMONIAL

Two years ago, I was moving out of my San Francisco apartment. I'd spilled red wine on the bedroom carpet and had planned to hire a professional cleaner, but I ran out of time and decided to take care of it myself. My boyfriend—now husband—came back from the store with a heavy-duty carpet-cleaning product. I never bought toxic stuff like that—I care about the environment and always bought biodegradable cleaning and bath products—but I was in a rush and this was what I had at hand.

He warned me to wear gloves when I used it, but I was too busy to bother. I never could have imagined what a life-changing decision that would be.

When I finished cleaning the carpet, I noticed my knuckles were bright red. I scrubbed my hands, slapped on some lotion and forgot about it. Then, about a week later, I noticed my hands were stiffening up and swelling. I'd wake up in the middle of the night and my hands would be "asleep." I went to a doctor, who diagnosed carpel tunnel syndrome, told me I was totally stressed and should pop a Valium and calm down. Eventually, I'd "be fine." I was about to embark on a 6-month trip around the world, so I was relieved to get the news.

Unfortunately, while I was traveling, my condition worsened. In each country I visited, I went to different doctors or healers to see if they could diagnose the problem and treat me. No one knew what was wrong with me.

Four months into my trip, the swelling started moving up my forearms, and the skin on my face and neck started tightening. I couldn't lift or hold anything tight or make a fist. When I got to England, I went to an acupuncturist, who diagnosed rheumatoid arthritis. I felt a mixture of shock and disbelief. I rushed back to the States and went to a specialist, who confirmed the diagnosis. She explained my prognosis—which wasn't pretty—put me on steroids, and told me I'd be on medication the rest of my life.

Then, as if it wasn't bad enough, I went to another doctor, who diagnosed scleroderma, a little-known autoimmune disease that causes the body to produce too much collagen. Ultimately, if it spreads to the lungs, it's fatal. I was told there was no cure.

I refused to accept that. I wanted to get to the root problem and be well again. So I began doing research into alternative medicine and healing through foods. I learned that that 80 to 90% of patients with scleroderma came down with the disease after some kind of chemical exposure. The lightbulb finally went off for me. I could trace everything I was experiencing back to that carpet cleaner.

Unlike the Western physicians I'd seen, the Eastern practitioners I found gave me hope that there was a way back to health. If I believed that my scleroderma was chemically induced, I needed to do something *to purge the toxins from my body. It was time to take my treatment into my own hands.*

I started by doing the Winter Wake-Up Cleanse with Adina and cut out all caffeine and alcohol. I could feel my symptoms easing a bit, but it still wasn't enough to purge the concentration of toxic chemicals from my body. So I went to Florida and checked myself into the Hippocrates Health Institute—a holistic healing facility in West Palm Beach that uses food as medicine. For 28 days, I ate nothing but a raw-foods diet. I took supplements such as chlorella and enzymes and did a variety of activities designed to pull the toxins from my body, including enemas, massage, saunas, hydrotherapy plunges and foot baths.

To be fully healed, I knew I had to have my mind in the right place as well. So I meditated throughout the day, visualizing myself being in optimal health. I saw myself as a healthy person—period. In the end, I believe that that was as important as the cleansing itself. I was also fortunate to have the loving support of the man who is now my husband. I don't know if I could have had the strength without him. It's great to have loved ones standing by you when you're facing a battle like this.

As my body finally shed the toxins, my skin began to loosen, I got my energy back and I regained flexibility in my hands as the swelling subsided. Now, I'm healthier than I've been in my entire life.

Two years ago, I had a chemically-induced life-threatening disease. One year later, I was feeling great and was pregnant with my first child. And today, I have a happy, healthy baby in my arms.

These days, I'm completely conscious of what I put in my body and on my body—the same goes for my baby. After seeing what I went through, members of my family completely "greened" their homes as well. We went through and replaced all their chemical products with biodegradable alternatives. It's so much easier than people might think—there are some great products out there.

I'm living proof that we can heal and protect our bodies through cleansing, meditation and making wise choices in the products we use.

When enough people experience the benefits of the alternatives, the alternatives will become the mainstream.

GOING GREEN

The recipes in this chapter include eco- and body-friendly products for the home and body. There are also a wide range of "green" substitutes available at grocery and health-food stores. Green products have come a long way just since 2000, so if you tried them a while ago and weren't impressed, give them another shot!

Three good brands to try are Shaklee, Seventh Generation and Mrs. Meyer's Clean Day, which offer safe alternatives to chemically laden products.

Special Equipment*

* 16-ounce glass pump bottle or dispenser
* 1-ounce travel-size spray bottle
* 1/8-ounce travel-size leakproof glass jar
* 4-ounce glass pump dispenser
* Two 16-ounce glass leakproof jars
* 40-ounce spray bottle

RECIPES

NOTE: All specialty ingredients can be found at health-food stores. The washing soda and borax can be found at health food, some grocery and some home-improvement stores.

---

* *Stores such as Bed Bath & Beyond and The Container Store carry these containers.*

Body

PEARLY-WHITES TOOTHPASTE

Makes 1 application

The abrasives in the baking soda and the antibacterial properties of the hydrogen peroxide in this recipe are a powerful antiplaque combination. Your teeth will feel as if you've just left the dentist's office. Food-grade hydrogen peroxide comes in a different concentration from regular hydrogen peroxide and is available at health-food stores. This recipe should be made 1 application at a time. Make sure you spit; don't swallow.

1 tablespoon baking soda
½ teaspoon food-grade hydrogen peroxide
2 drops peppermint or wintergreen extract

Directions: Mix all the ingredients together into a paste in the palm of your hand or a small cup. Apply ½ teaspoon to toothbrush and begin brushing. Apply another ½ teaspoon and continue brushing. Repeat until you've brushed all your teeth.

LOVE-YOUR-BODY SOAP

Makes 8 ounces

This soap will leave you feeling smooth and squeaky clean. You can use it on your hands, face or entire body. Create a few different versions, using different essential oils, to match your moods on different days. I love lavender when I'm stressed, ylang-ylang when I'm feeling sensual, and eucalyptus or peppermint when I need a pick-me-up.

1 cup unscented liquid glycerin soap (available at local health-food stores)
4–6 drops essential oil of your choice
16-ounce glass pump bottle or dispenser

Directions: Pour soap into a medium bowl. Add essential oil drops. Mix gently until oils are incorporated. Pour soap into a pump or squeeze bottle to store. Use as needed.

SKIN-LOVING MOISTURIZERS

Want to get supple, soft skin without slathering on chemicals? Just rub a little jojoba, almond, olive or coconut oil into your skin after a bath or shower and get a natural glow!

OOH-LA-LA NATURAL SCENTS

Makes 1 ounce

Our taste in perfume is as unique as our taste in clothing. One size doesn't fit all, and our preferences may change with our moods. This recipe helps you create healthy, personalized scents that won't leave toxins on your skin or in the air. Spritz throughout the day on your pulse points and your hair. Some essential oils have more powerful scents than others, so start conservatively and gradually add more oil, as needed, to get to the level of scent you desire. Create different versions to match your mood or experiment in combining oils to develop your own signature scent.

1 ounce purified water
4 drops essential oil of your choice
1-ounce travel-size spray bottle

Directions: Add water and essential oil to spray bottle. Shake gently to combine, and start spritzing!

KISS-ME LIP BALM

Makes 1/8 ounce

Many commercially produced lip balms have petroleum bases, which actually dry out your lips. This lip balm is easy to make, tastes good and moisturizes your lips. Stevia is a powerful natural sweetener found in plants, so get ready for your sweetest kiss yet!

1/8 ounce shea butter
Small pinch of stevia
1 drop peppermint, lavender or rose essential oil
1/8 ounce leakproof glass jar

Directions: Mix shea butter, stevia and essential oil together in a small cup. Spoon into jar. Pucker up, spread on your lips and re-seal.

BODY-FRIENDLY BATH SALTS

Makes enough for 1 bath

Epsom salts leave your skin feeling soft and are great for pulling lactic acid or toxins out of muscles. Use a rejuvenating essential oil like juniper or eucalyptus if you want a pick-me-up before a night on the town; add sandalwood or patchouli to set a sensual mood for the evening; or go with lavender to unwind before bedtime.

1 cup Epsom salts
4 drops essential oil of your choice

Directions: Draw bath. Add Epsom salts and essential oils to water. Stir to dissolve salt, and then step into your bath.

"OH, MY ACHING DOGS" FOOT BATH

Makes 1 treatment

After a long day on your feet, this is a wonderfully rejuvenating foot soak. The rosemary and sage improve circulation, the cloves help relieve pain, and the juniper berries kill bacteria that cause odors and pull toxins from the body.

1 cup boiling water
10–12 juniper berries
5 whole cloves
1 teaspoon dried rosemary
1 teaspoon dried sage
2 gallons very warm water

Directions: Pour the first 5 ingredients into a mug and steep, like a tea, for 10 minutes. Pour the 2 gallons of water, as warm as you can bear it, into a bucket large enough to stick your feet in. Add the steeped spice mixture. Ease feet into the bath and soak for at least 10 minutes.

SWEET CARESS MASSAGE OILS

Makes 4 ounces

Your skin will drink this up! Add an essential oil that matches the mood you're trying to create. Jasmine or ylang-ylang are said to stoke romantic flames, rosewood or chamomile are relaxing, and bergamot or orange are reenergizing.

4 ounces jojoba oil
3 drops essential oil of your choice
4-ounce glass dispenser

Directions: Pour jojoba oil into a small bowl. Add essential oils and stir to incorporate. Transfer to dispenser to store for later use.

NEW SKIN SALT SCRUB

Makes 16 ounces

This is a great natural exfoliant—your skin will feel as smooth as a baby's bottom. The ground ginger is stimulating and warming to the body and the almond oil is calming and sweet. Add a few drops of your favorite essential oil if you want to spice it up a bit.

1 cup coarse sea salt
½ teaspoon ground ginger
½ cup jojoba oil
16-ounce leak-resistant jar

Directions: Mix ingredients together in a small bowl until combined. Transfer to jar. To use, wet the body and then gently rub about 1 tablespoon of the salt scrub into your skin in small circular motions. As salt disperses, repeat over all areas of the body (avoiding eyes, mouth and genitalia). Rinse off in a shower or bath, and then towel dry. Store unused salt scrub out of direct sunlight.

Home

STREAK-FREE WINDOW CLEANER

Makes 24 ounces

Warn the birds, because your windows will be so clean they'll pose a flight hazard. Drying the windows with newspaper rather than rags eliminates lint on the glass.

1 cup white vinegar
2 cups warm water
Clean rags
Sections of newspaper

Directions: Mix water and vinegar together in a bucket. Soak and lightly wring rag in the water–vinegar combo. Wash window with rag. Starting from top to bottom, use pieces of newspaper to dry the glass.

MOP-IT-UP ALL-PURPOSE CLEANER

Makes 5 applications

This cleaner has the eco seal of approval from bare feet and crawling babies. The washing soda, a more alkaline version of common baking soda, is great at fighting tough stains. It's biologically friendly but could still irritate sensitive skin, so be sure to use gloves. The lavender serves as a great disinfectant, and it smells wonderful too.

2 teaspoons borax
2 teaspoons washing soda
¼ cup unscented liquid glycerin soap
¼ cup white vinegar
4 cups hot water
20 drops lavender oil
40-ounce glass bottle

Directions: Combine the borax, washing soda and soap in a bucket or spray bottle, depending on what you'll be using it for. Pour in vinegar and hot water to dissolve the minerals, and then add the essential oil. If you store it in a spray bottle, shake the bottle before each use.

BLEACH-ALTERNATIVE BATHROOM AND KITCHEN CLEANER

Makes 1 application

You can shed the rubber gloves with this cleaner—no chemicals to leach into the body and dry the skin.

½ cup washing soda
1 cup warm water

Directions: Mix ingredients together in a bucket or bowl. Scrub area to be cleaned with a sponge or scrub brush. Reapply, as needed.

OUT, DAMNED SPOT!

The cleaning agent perchloroethylene, or "perc," used by most dry cleaners, can cause adverse health effects on the nervous system, including dizziness, fatigue, headaches, sweating, incoordination, and unconsciousness. Long-term exposure has been connected to liver and kidney damage. So look for dry cleaners who use body-friendly solutions such as wet cleaning or liquid carbon dioxide solvents.

COLORFAST LAUNDRY DETERGENT

Makes 2 cups

One of the greatest polluters of U.S. waterways is laundry detergent, given the large amounts we use and the toxins found in most commercial brands. This eco-friendly alternative is gentler on your clothing and the Earth and still gets the job done with a fraction of the amount of detergent used in commercial solutions.

1 cup grated Ivory bar soap
½ cup washing soda
½ cup borax
16-ounce glass jar

Directions: Mix the ingredients together in a small bowl until all have been incorporated. Transfer to a resealable container. Use 1 tablespoon for a light load of laundry and 2 tablespoons for a heavy load of laundry. A little goes a long way!

Cleanse-Boosting Activities

Clean House

To purge your home of harmful chemicals, go around and pull out all of the cleaning products under your kitchen and bathroom sinks. Then do the same with your medicine cabinets and vanities: Take out the personal-care products and put them on the counter. Look at the list of ingredients on each product and keep a running list of the different chemicals. Then ask yourself how often you and your family are exposed to all those chemicals. Pick three to five from the list and do a little Internet research on each of them—you may be unpleasantly surprised by what you learn. Before you get overwhelmed or discouraged, think about which of these products has green, biodegradable alternatives and consider testing some. Even if you replaced one, three or five toxic products in your home, you'd be reducing your exposure to harmful chemicals and creating a cleaner, safer home.

WATCHING WHAT WE USE TO COOK AND STORE FOOD

When it comes to preparing and storing food, we can protect our and our family's health by getting rid of nonstick pans, aluminum pans and baking sheets, and plastic storage containers.

- Studies have shown that the perfluorooctanoic acid used to make nonstick coatings is showing up in human bloodstreams. The Environmental Protection Agency has labeled the chemical a "likely carcinogen" and asked that the chemical be phased out of production by 2015. Use a little elbow grease and switch to steel, cast-iron or copper pans.

- Some researchers have labeled aluminum a neurotoxin and linked it to Alzheimer's disease, so toss out those aluminum pans and baking sheets and replace them with steel or cast iron.

- Toxins connected to cancer and endocrine problems leach out of the plastic storage containers we use into the food or liquid they're holding, so consider trading in the plastic for glass.

Spread the Love

The lotions, soaps, scrubs and oils for the body included in this chapter make great body-friendly, eco-friendly gifts for friends and family. Any occasion is the right time to spread the love! Search online or at local stores for fun jars or bottles in which to package your homemade concoctions. You can decorate the lids or containers with paint or labels to personalize the gift and make it even more special. (Don't forget to mention that it's all natural and made with love!)

Make a Difference Outside Your Home

Like many of my clients, you may feel a sense of responsibility to be kinder and gentler to yourself and to the planet after doing a dietary cleanse. Here's a list of easy things you can do on a daily basis that will have a positive impact on the Earth and your spirit:

✴ Buy a canteen or glass bottle that you can continue to refill with water, rather than buying little plastic water bottles that are tossed after one use. You'll be conserving resources, taking pressure off the landfills and reducing your intake of the chemicals that leach out of plastics.

✳ Bring your own reusable bags to the grocery store. If you forget, ask for paper rather than plastic and reuse that paper bag several times before recycling it.

✳ Buy a stainless-steel sealable mug and bring that to your local tea or coffee shop rather than using the store's paper or polystyrene cups. If you leave your cup at home and need to use a disposable one, use that cup for refills rather than throwing it out after one use.

✳ If you hear or read about a green product that isn't in your local market, ask the store manager to start carrying it. Demand dictates supply: If we ask for the products we want, many stores will consider putting them on their shelves.

✳ If you get food to go on a regular basis, don't use the plastic forks, spoons or knives they offer. Health-food stores carry reusable bamboo cutlery sets, or you can stock your desk or bag with a set of stainless utensils from home.

✳ Buy local organic foods. You'll be supporting the green economy, reducing your intake of chemically treated foods, and cutting down on the fuel used and emissions released into the environment when food is transported long distances.

BREAKING A CLEANSE

In this chapter, we talk about how to break a cleanse. When you've eaten clean foods to detox your body, you need to be mindful about how you reintroduce foods so that you don't shock your system, particularly if you've chosen cleanses other than the One-Day Wonder or the Three-Day Face-Lift. Then, after we get through the process of breaking a cleanse, we have a choice to make: Do we want to maintain the high we feel and keep nurturing our body, or will we return to a diet that might not have been supporting our health?

You may not be ready to become a raw-foodist and you may not want to be a vegetarian, but introducing cleansing, alkaline foods into your everyday diet is essential. It all comes down to knowing the good from the bad apples and striking a balance.

The more raw, vegetarian food you can build into your ongoing diet, the better, and it would be ideal to eliminate the Dirty Baker's Dozen (see page 2) entirely. I'm a huge advocate of that, but I also know that eating differently over the long haul is an evolution for most of us. So I'd rather encourage you to take whatever steps you can to stay on the path toward healthier eating than promote one stringent approach that you might decide you can't stick with. Start where you are and move forward from there.

FOOD COMBINATIONS

The standard American diet that traditionally includes protein, starch and vegetables in one meal is tough on the digestive tract. Each of those foods digests at different rates, and the body works overtime sorting it all out. Combining foods properly is a great habit to get into over the long term, and it's especially important when you're breaking a cleanse. Follow these easy tips for the week after a cleanse—and consider making them a part of your regular meal planning:

- Eat proteins with sprouts and vegetables.
- Eat starches with sprouts and vegetables.
- Avoid mixing starches and proteins.
- Eat fruit alone.

Universal Tips for Breaking a Cleanse

How you break a cleanse and reintroduce foods into your diet varies by cleanse: The more stringent the cleanse, the more slowly you should reintroduce different foods. These pointers apply to breaking any of the cleanses:

✳ We don't need to eat as much to sustain ourselves as we think we do. Eat small portions, eat slowly, and chew your food thoroughly.

✳ Drink a green juice every day, or make a green soup or smoothie. (Make that a part of your long-term routine as well!)

✳ Take probiotics and digestive enzymes to promote the growth of good intestinal bacteria and aid in digestion.

✳ Stick with eating organic products.

* Avoid commercial dairy and processed grains, sugars and fats.

* Eat when you're hungry; avoid eating to cope with boredom or stress.

* Notice whether your sense of taste has changed. After a cleanse, many people don't crave or enjoy foods that undermine their health. They find that they can (and want to!) kick the habit of eating certain foods.

* Pay attention to your digestion/elimination and your energy levels as you introduce foods. You may find that you're sensitive to some foods.

* If you resume consumption of alcohol or caffeine, do it very slowly. Their effects may be greatly increased, particularly after the more rigorous cleanses.

* If you want to introduce meat proteins, start with lightly steamed fish, free-range organic eggs or free-range organic chicken.

Breaking a Stringent Cleanse

If you've just completed the Urban Revitalizer, Winter Wake-Up or Green Buzz cleanses, it's important to reintroduce foods even more carefully. You'll have just been on a regimen of alkaline, easy-to-digest liquid nutrition, so it's best to start off with raw vegetables, fruits, sprouts, salads, seeds, nuts and cold-pressed oils, and then transition to eating cooked vegetables, grains and legumes before deciding if you're going to return to cooked proteins.

To make it easier for you to choose the right foods to eat, I recommend taking the following phased approach to breaking those three cleanses:

	Eat Fruit, Salads, Raw and Cooked Vegetables, and Vegetable Broths	Eat Select Meals from the Laughing Buddha* and "Some Like it Raw"* Cleanses
Urban Revitalizer	2 days	2 days
Winter Wake-Up	3 days	3 days
Green Buzz	3 days	3 days

Look for recipes from the chapters on cleanses with an asterisk next to the names. They'll be the best alternatives to start with.

Following the program above may sound like "the cleanse after the cleanse," but believe me, the range of flavors and textures will taste heavenly and your body will thank you for the slow reintroduction of different foods.

Purging the Pantry

If you have an experience like that of many of my clients, then once you've completed a cleanse, you may want to start eating differently on a regular basis. For many of us that means learning to plan meals differently. Choosing and preparing different foods is like learning a new language. Examining what's currently stocking your kitchen, flagging the bad things and exploring alternatives is a great way to begin. As you look through your refrigerator and cupboards, consider the following substitutions and recommendations:

Items to Purge from the Pantry	Substitutions
Meats with antibiotics and hormones, farm-raised fish	• If you want meat protein, choose organic chicken and wild-caught fish. • If you're going to eat red meat, have it once in a while and make sure it's grass-fed and organic.

(continued)

Items to Purge from the Pantry	Substitutions
	• Alternative sources of protein include sprouted beans, nuts, seeds and legumes; blue-green algae; and açaí, goji and Incan berries. See recipes from the cleansing chapters that have these ingredients.
Processed grains and flours	• Use whole grains such as quinoa, amaranth, spelt, millet and wild rice. • In place of bleached white flour, try substituting spelt flour, millet flour, quinoa flour, buckwheat flour or chickpea flour. • Healthier substitutions for pasta include quinoa, spaghetti squash, spiralized zucchini and spelt or brown-rice pasta.
Processed sugars and sweeteners	• Stevia, raw honey, raw agave, grade B maple syrup and yacon are great substitutes for processed sugar. They've got varying degrees of sweetness, so check a cookbook or online to determine the ratio for substitutions.
Cookies, candy, cakes; refined-grain breads and crackers	• Many health-food stores and some grocery stores carry a selection of sprouted-grain or whole-grain breads and raw crackers that don't clog the system (look for the bread in the refrigerated section). • Eat fresh and dried fruit in place of candy, cookies and other sweets. • Enjoy raw cookies or desserts in moderation. You can find them in many health-food stores.
Commercial dairy products	• Nut milks and coconut milk • Nut cheeses • Raw, unpasteurized cheese (in moderation) • Raw, unpasteurized yogurt (in moderation) • Goat kefir
Refined oils	• Don't heat oils. If you choose to, it's best to use cold-pressed olive or coconut oil. • Raw, cold-pressed oils are medicinal. They have essential fatty acids our bodies need to thrive—as long as they stay raw. I recommend

(*continued*)

Items to Purge from the Pantry	Substitutions
	flax oil, Udo's oil, hemp oil, coconut oil and cold-pressed olive oil for things like salad dressing (flax, hemp and Udo's oils should be refrigerated and never heated).
Sweetened juices and sodas	• Choose 100% juice or make your own. • Mix naturally fizzy water (such as San Pellegrino) and 100% juice for a healthy alternative to sodas.
White potatoes	• Sweet potatoes, yams and winter squash are better alternatives.

Restocking the Larder

Once you've purged the pantry, it's time to restock with healthy essentials. The suggestions below are adapted from my studies at The Natural Gourmet Cookery School in New York City. The majority are used in recipes from the different cleanses, so flip back through the chapters and test some of those recipes. As you experiment with these ingredients, you'll get more and more comfortable creating meals with them.

NOTE: With the exception of the dried legumes, it's better to buy in smaller quantities rather than in bulk to keep the ingredients fresh.

LEGUMES	SEEDS	CONDIMENTS
• Beans (adzuki, black, cannellini, mung, pinto, or turtle) • Chickpeas • Lentils	• Flax • Hemp • Pumpkin • Sesame • Sunflower • Chia	• Capers • Chutney • Dijon mustard • Kimchee • Miso (chickpea and barley) • Nut butters (raw)
WHOLE GRAINS		• Olives
• Amaranth • Brown rice • Buckwheat (soba) • Millet • Quinoa • Wild rice	**OILS (COLD-PRESSED)** • Coconut • Flaxseed • Ghee • Hemp • Olive	• Pickled ginger • Shoyu (in moderation) • Spices and herbs • Sun-dried tomatoes • Tahini • Tamari (in moderation)
PROCESSED GRAINS	• Pumpkin • Udo's	• Wasabi
• Buckwheat flour • Chickpea flour • Millet flour • Quinoa pasta • Spelt flour/pasta	**DRIED FRUIT** • Apricots • Cranberries • Dates	**VINEGAR** • Apple cider • Balsamic • Brown rice • Red wine • Umeboshi
NUTS (RAW)	• Figs • Mango • Papaya • Raisins	**SEAWEED**
• Almonds • Brazil nuts • Coconut • Filberts • Macadamia • Pecans • Pine nuts • Walnuts • Cashews	**THICKENING AGENTS** • Agar-agar • Arrowroot powder • Flaxseed • Kuzu • Psyllium husks • Tapioca	• Arame • Dulse • Hijiki • Kombu • Nori • Wakame **TEAS** • Chamomile • Dandelion

(continued)

LEGUMES	SEEDS	CONDIMENTS
FRESH VEGETABLES	**BAKING PRODUCTS**	• Decaf chai blends
• Local, organic and seasonal	• Baking soda	• Ginger
	• Nonaluminum baking powder	• Licorice root
		• Milk thistle
		• Mint
		• Nettles
		• Red clover blossom
		• Rooibos
		• Tulsi

Follow the "pHood" Chart

Getting a handle on the relative alkalinity and acidity of different foods is another helpful way to approach meal planning after a cleanse. Acidic foods aren't necessarily bad in and of themselves, but consuming too many of them over long periods of time does affect our health. We need both acidic and alkaline foods in our diet, but our diet should be predominantly alkaline. It's all about balance.

The chart below shows where different foods fall on the pH spectrum. Ideally, the bulk of your diet will come from the alkaline side of the chart. Think of it this way: Try to build more fresh vegetables, sprouted grains, seeds, nuts, whole grains, fruits and blue-green algae into your diet. The more sprouted, the better!

Highly Alkaline ⬅━━━━━━━➡			Highly Acidic
GREENS • All vegetables (except those listed elsewhere) • Grasses • Leafy greens • Sea vegetables • Sprouts **HEALTHY FATS AND OILS** • Avocado • Borage • Coconut • Evening primrose • Fish • Flax • Hemp • Olive • Udo's **OTHER** • Alkalized, purified water • Bee pollen • Green powders (such as chlorella, spirulina and other blue-green algae) • Himalayan and Celtic sea salts	**LOW-SUGAR FRUITS** • Avocados • Grapefruit • Lemons • Limes • Tomatoes **SPROUTED NUT AND SEED MILKS** • Almond • Brazil nuts • Hazelnuts • Hemp seed • Pecan • Sesame seed **OTHER VEGETABLES AND HERBS** • Artichoke • Asparagus • Cabbage • Celery • Celery root • Eggplant • Garlic • Green peas • Hearts of palm • Herbs (fresh, dry) • Onion • Organic spices • Radish	**COOKED/STEAMED VEGETABLES STARCHES** • Beets • Carrots • Parsnips • Pumpkin • Rutabaga • Sprouted grains • Sprouted legumes • Sweet potatoes • Yams **HIGH-SUGAR FRUITS** (All fruits not listed as low-sugar) **SWEETENERS/ FLAVORINGS** • Stevia **FRESHWATER FISH** (Eat sparingly) **HERBAL TEAS** **SPROUTED NUTS AND SEEDS** • Almond • Brazil nuts • Cacao • Hazelnuts • Hemp seeds • Macadamia nuts	**PROCESSED FOODS** • Canned foods • Microwaved foods • Preservatives **ALL ANIMAL PRODUCTS STORED GRAINS/ RISEN DOUGH/ FUNGAL STARCH** • Rye bread • White bread • White potatoes • Whole-grain bread • Whole-meal bread **FUNGI** • Cashews • Corn • Mushrooms • Peanuts • Pistachios **FATS** • Butter • Heated oils • Margarine **SWEETS AND STRONG ACID** • Agave

(continued)

Highly Alkaline ⟵——————————⟶ Highly Acidic		
SPROUTED GRAINS (USE SPARINGLY) • Buckwheat • Quinoa • Spelt	**SPROUTED NUTS AND SEEDS** • Pecans • Pumpkinseeds • Sesame seeds • Walnuts	**SWEETS AND STRONG ACID** • Alcohol • Artificial sweeteners • Caffeine • Honey (raw and processed) • Refined chocolate • Refined sugars and corn syrups • Vinegar • Yeast

Super Supplements

The following list of superfoods and supplements are excellent sources of things that your body needs to thrive, such as protein, enzymes, chlorophyll, minerals and vitamins. Experiment with making them part of your daily routine for a boost of nutrients, to alkalize the body and to help sustain a healthy digestive tract. They'll help you keep the glow and maintain the energy boost you get from a cleanse.

Superfood/Supplement	Benefit
Açaí or goji berries/juice	Rich in antioxidants, essential fatty acids, fiber and flavonoids—all tied to preventing cancer and hypertension
Bee pollen (unless you're allergic to bee stings)	High in protein and vitamin B_{12}; boosts immunity

(continued)

Superfood/Supplement	Benefit
Blue-green algae (such as chlorella and spirulina) and green cereal grasses	Among the richest whole-food proteins in the world. They're dense in chlorophyll, which has antioxidant and anti-inflammatory properties; clean the blood and are good for mental health; and pull toxins from the liver and digestive tract. Chlorella, in particular, is packed with nutrients and helps pull toxic metals and chemicals from the body.
Digestive enzymes	Bolster digestive enzymes in the body, assisting in proper digestion
Flax, hemp, pumpkin, borage, evening primrose and fish oils	Great for the skin; provide essential fatty acids, which decrease inflammation, improve brain function, and nourish the heart and eyes
Lecithin	Assists in the breakdown of fats and cholesterol, supporting heart health; cleanses the liver and kidneys; reduces inflammation
Maca	This highly nutritious root from Peru has been found to boost endurance, alleviate stress and balance hormones in the body.
MSM (methylsulfonylmethane)	Maintains skin elasticity; reduces inflammation; promotes healthy hair and nails
Probiotics	Introduce healthy bacteria to the digestive tract to fuel proper digestion.
Sprouts	Sprouted seeds, nuts, grains and legumes are the greatest source of protein in the vegetable kingdom. In addition, they're chock-full of vitamins, minerals, enzymes and essential fatty acids.
Tocotrienols	Excellent source of vitamin E, which is great for the skin. High in antioxidants that help prevent cancer, reduce cholesterol and stimulate the immune system.
Vitamin C	Helps repair body tissues and fight disease and infections. It's particularly helpful in warding off colds. It's also an antioxidant that eliminates free radicals from the body.
Wheatgrass	Detoxifies the liver and blood, alkalizes the blood, and stimulates the thyroid, helping manage obesity and indigestion.

MEXICAN FIESTA

I created this chapter to be a celebration of healing foods. This Mexican feast is a recipe for looking at food differently, building community and reestablishing the ritual of preparing food with family and friends. Depending on what cleanse you choose, it's important to break your cleanse before trying these recipes to ensure that you don't introduce some foods too early.

Many of us have a very clear idea about what Mexican food is supposed to be like: Years of eating and seeing it have ingrained images and tastes in our minds. But this is a whole new enchilada! If you experiment with the recipes in this chapter, it will open your eyes to an entirely different, and healthier, way of enjoying south-of-the-border classics we know and love. I'll be honest with you—they won't taste or look exactly the same, but they're meals you'd be proud to serve at a dinner party.

I recommend soaking the beans and making the Oaxaca Tea Cookies in advance, but get the whole family or your crew of friends into the kitchen to take part in making the rest of the meal. Food tastes better when you're having fun making it together, and it's a great opportunity for everyone to start looking differently at food and how it can be prepared. So get ready to explore . . . *buen provecho!*

When to Do It

Have a Mexican fiesta if you want to revive the custom of eating together and celebrate food and abundance. Do it if you're excited by what you experienced during a cleanse and want to explore ways of cooking—or "uncooking"—differently on a regular basis.

What You'll See and Feel

Unlike some of the big family meals I had growing up, this feast won't make you have to loosen your waistband and take a nap afterward! You'll feel light and energized.

Special Equipment

* Food processor
* Blender
* Nut-milk bags (optional, if you choose to make your own nut milk—available at health-food stores)
* Parchment paper
* Dehydrator—optional, needed for one recipe

RECIPES

NOTE: Raw agave syrup, cacao nibs or powder, and almond milk are available at health-food stores and some grocery stores. Dulse powder, young coconuts and kombu are available at health-food stores and Asian markets. Chipotle chilies are available at Latin or specialty markets.

ZIPPY RAW CARROT SOUP

Makes 4 appetizer servings or 2 main-course servings

This raw spicy carrot soup is creamy and tangy, and a great appetizer or a delicious first course. I like to serve it in a martini glass to show off all the colors. You can make your own carrot juice or buy it at a juice bar or health-food store. My favorite garnishes for this soup are sprouts, chopped cucumber, avocado, cilantro and cayenne.

4 cups carrot juice, from approximately 24 carrots
1 large avocado, peeled and pitted
1 cucumber, peeled
1 red pepper, cut into small dice
½ teaspoon garlic, minced
1 tablespoon mint
1 teaspoon cilantro, chopped
½ jalapeño pepper, seeded and chopped
Pinch of Himalayan or Celtic sea salt
1 teaspoon cumin
1 teaspoon fresh lime juice, or more to taste
Optional garnishes: chopped herbs or sprouts

Directions: Pour the purchased carrot juice or juiced carrots into a blender. Add the avocado, cucumber, pepper, garlic, mint, cilantro, jalapeño, salt, cumin and lime juice. Blend until smooth. Add more lime juice and salt, and chopped herbs or sprouts, if desired. Serve in bowls.

SPICY BLACK BEAN SOUP

Makes 6 servings

Black beans are quite warming in the wintertime and good for your kidneys. You can pile all kinds of goodness on top of this easy-to-make soup. I like to have mine with the Green Spanish Rice and the Cucumber Salsa recipes included in this chapter!

1 cup dried black beans, soaked in water overnight
1 onion, cut into small dice
2 tablespoons cold-pressed extra virgin olive oil
3 large cloves garlic, peeled and minced
1/4 cup celery, cut into small dice
1/3 cup butternut or kabocha squash, cut into small dice
1 teaspoon fresh thyme, minced
1/2 teaspoon ground cumin
2 jalapeño chilies, seeded and minced
1 teaspoon puréed chipotle chili
1 cup chopped tomatoes
One 1-inch piece kombu
1 teaspoon Himalayan or Celtic sea salt, or more to taste

Directions: Drain the soaked beans and set aside. In a soup pot, sauté the onion in the oil until lightly brown for 5 minutes, and then add the garlic, celery, squash, thyme, cumin, jalapeño, and chipotle chili and sauté for another 5 minutes. Add the chopped tomatoes and the beans, kombu, and 2½ quarts water and bring to a boil. Lower heat and cook for 1 hour or more, depending on softness of beans. Discard the kombu piece and add salt in the last 10 minutes of cooking.

MEXICAN CAESAR SALAD WITH SPICY AVOCADO DRESSING

Makes 6 servings

Try this spin on your usual Caesar dressing. The dulse seaweed adds a little hint of smoke and deep flavor. Wash the leaves beforehand and keep them in the refrigerator until you serve them so your salad is extra crisp. Dress the salad just before serving.

SALAD

4 romaine lettuce heads, cut into bite-sized pieces
1 small jicama, peeled and cut into medium dice (like croutons)

Directions: In a large mixing bowl, toss the romaine lettuce and jicama with the dressing. You might want to use your hands so the dressing is evenly distributed.

DRESSING

3 avocados, peeled, pitted and cut into large dice
Juice of 2 limes
1 teaspoon jalapeño pepper sauce (beware, hot!)
1 teaspoon dulse powder
Several pinches of Himalayan or Celtic sea salt
Pinch of black pepper
1 clove garlic, minced

Directions: In a food processor, blend all ingredients until smooth. Mix dressing into salad.

GREEN SPANISH RICE WITH GREEN ONION AND AVOCADOS

Makes 6 servings

I've been eating Spanish rice since I was a kid, so it's always been a staple for me. This tasty twist on the original can be eaten alone as a meal. Try it on top of the tortilla pie and black bean soup.

1 tablespoon cold-pressed extra virgin olive oil
1 small onion, cut into small dice
1 clove garlic, minced
Pinch of Himalayan or Celtic sea salt, or more to taste
1 cup long-grain brown rice
2 cups vegetable broth or purified water
2 cups cilantro, chopped
1 green onion, green stalks only, chopped
Lime to taste
2 avocados, peeled and pitted

Directions: Heat oil in a 2-quart saucepan over medium heat. Add onion, garlic, and pinch of salt and sauté for 5 minutes. Add rice and broth or water. Bring to a boil and then lower to a simmer and cover and cook for 45 minutes, until water is absorbed. Let sit covered on stove for 10 minutes after done. Transfer to a mixing bowl and add cilantro, green onion, lime, and pinch of salt and toss well. Garnish with the avocados.

DIANARITA'S COLESLAW

Makes 4 servings

This became my favorite coleslaw on a summer day at my girlfriend Diana's house. I love the lime juice and creamy cumin sauce. Diana made it with yogurt; I made it vegan with a macadamia nut "sour cream." Delicioso!

SLAW

1 small head cabbage, cut into thin strips
1 small jicama, peeled and julienned

Directions: Put cabbage and jicama into a large bowl and mix in dressing.

DRESSING

1 cup macadamia nuts
¼ cup purified water
¼ cup lime juice
1 teaspoon ground cumin
⅛ teaspoon Himalayan or Celtic sea salt
½ cup cilantro, coarsely chopped, or more to taste

Directions: Process macadamia nuts in food processor until you get a fine meal consistency. Add water, lime juice, cumin, and salt and process until creamy. Toss creamy dressing over slaw and massage with your hands until it's completely coated with dressing. Toss in chopped cilantro.

10-MINUTE SPROUTED TORTILLA PIE
WITH CUCUMBER SALSA

Makes 3 servings

I concocted this pie while living in the Wasatch Mountains. It's
full of flavors and really easy to make. I love it because you can pile
just about anything on top. I like to serve this with the Zippy Raw
Carrot Soup and the Green Spanish Rice.

SPROUTED TORTILLA PIE

3 cups cooked white beans—rinsed, if canned
1 tablespoon cold-pressed extra virgin olive oil
3 large onions, cut into ribbons
2 poblano or Anaheim chilies, seeded and chopped
2 cloves garlic, peeled and minced
1/2 teaspoon ground cumin
Pinch of Himalayan or Celtic sea salt
6 sprouted-grain tortillas
3 avocados, peeled, pitted and sliced
Optional: green or Moroccan olives; lime wedges

Directions: Warm beans on stove in a medium pot and mash
with the back of a spoon into a soft paste. In a skillet, heat oil,
then add onions, chilies, garlic, cumin, and salt and sauté until
caramelized, at least 7 minutes. Add caramelized onions to
white bean mash and stir well. Remove from heat and season
with salt and pepper. Set aside, covered to keep warm. In a clean
skillet, toast tortillas on both sides until crisp. Spread three tortillas with some bean mixture, and top with onions, avocados

and optional olives. Squeeze a wedge of lime over the mixture, if
desired, and top with a second tortilla. Serve with Cucumber
Salsa.

CUCUMBER SALSA

6 ripe tomatoes
1 large cucumber, peeled and deseeded
¼ cup red onion, chopped
¼ cup cilantro, coarsely chopped
1 jalapeño, deseeded and minced
2 tablespoons fresh lime juice
Pinch of Himalayan or Celtic sea salt

Directions: Combine all ingredients in a bowl and serve with
Sprouted Tortilla Pie.

BEETS WITH ARUGULA AND PUMPKINSEEDS

Makes 4 servings

Beets clean the blood, moisten the intestines and are good for the
liver. I think they taste absolutely divine! This is a recipe you want
to keep on hand to nibble on all day.

6 large beets, well washed and cut into quarters
¼ cup apple cider vinegar
2 cups arugula
2 tablespoons toasted pumpkinseeds

Directions: Preheat oven to 400 degrees. Wrap each beet separately
in parchment paper. Roast in a pan in the oven for 35 to 40 min-

utes until tender. Remove from oven, let cool, and peel. Cut into slices, add vinegar and let marinate for 10 minutes. Toss beets in a bowl with arugula and toasted pumpkinseeds. Season with salt and pepper, as needed.

OAXACA TEA COOKIES

Makes 10 cookies

I love this recipe. The first time I tried these I could not believe it was a dehydrated cookie that wasn't filled with butter or sugar. Offer them up with a cup of hot tea and enjoy.

2 cups pecans, ground into fine meal
1 cup flaxseeds, ground into fine meal
1/4 teaspoon cinnamon
1 teaspoon Himalayan or Celtic sea salt
1/2 cup raisins, soaked in water for one hour
2 tablespoons raw honey
2 tablespoons cacao nibs
1 cup purified water
1/4 cup raw pistachios

Directions: Combine pecan meal, flax meal, cinnamon and salt in a mixing bowl. Transfer to a food processor and add raisins, honey and cacao. Start blending, adding water a little at a time, until you get thick heavy dough. Transfer dough back to mixing bowl and add pistachios. Shape the dough into a flat loaf on a board dusted with flaxseed meal. Put onto a Teflex sheet that's covered in parchment paper and dehydrate for 6 to 7 hours at 118 degrees, or longer if you'd like crunchier cookies.

MEXICAN MILK SHAKE

Makes 1 serving

This shake will take you to the moon. It's so damn good and so easy to make. Each of your guests can personalize their flavor with the variations included here, or come up with combinations of your own! Add six ice cubes or frozen fruit if you'd like a thicker milk shake. If you'd like faster preparation, substitute almond milk for the young coconut milk.

1 vanilla bean
1 cup water from a young coconut
3 tablespoons young coconut flesh, or more to taste (see instructions for opening a young coconut on page 160)
1 tablespoon raw cacao
2 pinches of cayenne
Pinch of Himalayan or Celtic sea salt

Directions: Split vanilla bean lengthwise, scrape out seeds into a blender, and discard the pod. Add water, coconut, cacao, cayenne, salt and your choice of optional ingredients (see below); blend until smooth.

Variations

Vanilla: Omit the cacao and cayenne, and add a soaked date or fig.

Mint Chip: Omit the cayenne, and add ½ teaspoon fresh, minced mint.

Tooty Fruity: Omit the cacao and cayenne, and add ¾ cup fresh or frozen fruit of your choice.

Activities

Set the Mood

When you throw your dinner party, make setting the table a family or group affair and get everyone involved. Have fun! Mix and match different plates or linens. Get a whole bunch of candles, gather some flowers or leaves, pick decorations that match the season. Feeling really creative? Paint or draw little works of art and put them next to each plate. If you have kids, let them choose which napkins you'll use and show them different fun ways to fold them. The possibilities are endless, but the goal is the same: to create a calm vibe before sitting down so that we can better appreciate one another and the food we're about to receive.

Express Gratitude

Sometimes it's easy to forget all the blessings in our lives and the abundance of choices we have. When you and your friends and loved ones are gathered together, getting ready to enjoy a great meal, it's a perfect time to pause to give thanks. Make it fun by playing this gratitude game before dinner:

* Give everyone something to write with and a piece of paper. (In the end, each person is going to write down something he or she is thankful for, but there's a twist.)

* Pick someone to get the ball rolling. Have that person write down one sentence on a piece of paper, saying what he or she is thankful for—it can be anything. He or she holds on to the piece of paper without reading the sentence aloud (yet), and doesn't show it to anyone except the person on his or her left.

* Then that person to the left writes down a sentence on his or her own piece of paper—building off what the other per-

son wrote—describing something he or she is thankful for. This person does not read the sentence aloud, and only shows it to the person on his or her left.

✳ Continue around the table until everyone has written a sentence.

✳ Once everyone has a sentence in hand, have the first person who wrote a sentence read his aloud. Then the person who wrote the second sentence reads hers, then the third, and so on.

In the end you'll have a homemade grace to go with your homemade meal—and hopefully a few laughs to boot. P.S. Speaking of gratitude, don't forget to kiss the cook(s)!

END ON A HIGH NOTE

Doing a cleanse and looking at food differently is like traveling to a foreign country: You step out of your familiar environment, explore, learn, and look at things with open eyes and a fresh perspective. It's my hope that doing any of the cleanses in this book created that experience for you, and that you're inspired to continue being an evolutionary in all parts of your life.

These themes that I wove in throughout the book brought me this far and continue to light my path along the way. They may be uplifting reminders on your journey as well:

Choose.

Have faith.

Keep it light.

Be grateful.

Unplug.

Avoid judgment.

Think differently.

Be still.

Laugh out loud.

Pull yourself out.

Follow your own rhythm.

Reconnect.

Give more.

RESOURCES

Anatomy of the Spirit: The Seven Stages of Power and Healing, Caroline Myss, PhD

Ask and It Is Given: Learning to Manifest Your Desires, Esther and Jerry Hicks

Book of Whole Meals: A Seasonal Guide to Assembling Balanced Vegetarian Breakfasts, Lunches and Dinners, Annemarie Colbin

Diet for a New America, John Robbins

Eating for Beauty, David Wolfe

Esoteric Anatomy: The Body as Consciousness, Bruce Burger

Heal Your Body A–Z, Louise Hay

The Healing Power of Chlorophyll from Plant Life, Bernard Jensen

Healing with Whole Foods: Asian Traditions and Modern Nutrition, Paul Pitchford

Healthful Cuisine, Anna Maria Clement

The Hippocrates Diet and Health Program, Ann Wigmore

How to Get Well: Dr. Airola's Handbook of Natural Healing, Paavo Airola

JillPettijohn.com

Jubb's Cell Rejuvenation—Colloidal Biology: A Symbiosis, David Jubb

The pH Miracle: Balance Your Diet, Reclaim Your Health, Robert O. Young, PhD, and Shelley Redford Young

Prakruti: Your Ayurvedic Constitution, Dr. Robert E. Svoboda

Rainbow Green Live-Food Cuisine, Gabriel Cousens, MD

The Self-Healing Cookbook: Whole Foods to Balance Body, Mind and Moods, Kristina Turner

Sprout for the Love of Everybody, Viktoras Kulvinskas

Staying Healthy with Nutrition, Elson Haas, MD

Vital Creations, Chad Sarno

INDEX